MEDICAL THINGS EXPLAINED

MTE

by Stacie the PA

Heart Failure 101:

A Patient's Complete Guide to Symptoms, Treatments, and Prevention

By Stacie the PA

For permission requests, contact:
Medical Things Explained
Email: *medicalthingsexplained@gmail.com*

ISBN: 978-1-970376-02-9

Printed in the United States of America
First Edition, 2025

Cover design and layout by **Stacie the PA™**
Published by **Medical Things Explained / Stacie the PA / Bowker**

Disclaimer

This book is for educational purposes only and is not intended to replace professional medical advice, diagnosis, or treatment.

Heart disease can be **life-threatening** and requires medical evaluation and ongoing care by qualified healthcare professionals.

Always seek the advice of your physician, cardiologist, or other licensed healthcare provider with any questions you may have about your symptoms, diagnosis, or treatment plan.

Never disregard professional medical advice or delay seeking it because of something you have read in this book.

If you think you may be experiencing a heart attack, stroke, or other medical emergency, call **911** or your local emergency number immediately.

Medication names, brand names, and supplement examples are provided for patient understanding only and do not represent endorsement by the author.

Readers should consult their healthcare team before beginning any new medication, supplement, diet, exercise program, or lifestyle change.

Some links or products mentioned may appear on the author's Amazon page as part of an affiliate partnership.If a purchase is made through those links, the author may receive a small commission at no additional cost to the reader. These partnerships help support future patient education materials.

Acknowledgement and Dedication

I would like to extend my heartfelt gratitude to the many healthcare professionals I have had the privilege of learning from and working alongside throughout my career.

From teachers and professors who built the foundation of my medical education to the clinicians and support staff who bring compassion to every patient encounter—you have each shaped my understanding of medicine and humanity in lasting ways.

During my training at Duke University Hospital, I had the extraordinary opportunity to rotate through cardiovascular surgery—assisting in open-heart procedures and caring for patients in the cardiac ICU.

The pace was intense, the teamwork seamless, and the experience unforgettable.

Later, as a practicing Physician Assistant, I briefly returned to open-heart surgery to cover a colleague's leave. It was so amazing to watch a still heart return to beating again.

*To my colleagues in medicine—**physicians, physician assistants, nurse practitioners, nurses, anesthetists, pharmacists, therapists, social workers, and pharmacists**—thank you for your knowledge, mentorship, and shared commitment to helping patients heal.*

To the administrative staff, technicians, and ICU teams who make complex care possible, your work is deeply valued and never unseen.

Your skill, teamwork, and dedication continue to inspire me.

This book—and the entire Patient Education 101 Series—is dedicated to all of you who serve, teach, and lead with heart.

Thank you for reminding me every day that medicine, at its best, is both a science and an art.

How to Use This Book

I've met many patients who left their first office visit (doesn't matter what speciality) more confused than comforted. This book is for you — to help you understand what's happening and feel in control–Stacie the PA.

- This book is meant to be a **guide you can write in, underline, and revisit.**

- You'll find short explanations, simple drawings, and checklists.
- You'll also see areas for notes throughout the book — blank sections where you can jot down thoughts, questions, or information from your provider.

For example:

- Write down your blood pressure numbers
- Keep track of new symptoms or medication changes
- Record what your doctor or nurse explains during visits

✎ **Notes:**

Warning Signs of Heart Failure Flare-Up

- Sudden shortness of breath, especially at night or when lying down
- Weight gain of 2–3 pounds overnight or 5 pounds in a week
- New swelling in your feet, ankles, or belly
- Needing more pillows to breathe comfortably
- Unusual fatigue or confusion

Call your medical provider right away — early treatment can prevent hospitalization.

Warning Signs of Dangerous Heart Rhythm

- Heart racing or fluttering that won't stop
- Dizziness or fainting
- Chest pressure or shortness of breath
- Feeling lightheaded or like you might pass out

If symptoms are severe or last longer than a few minutes, **call 911**.

While Waiting for Help

1. **Sit or lie down** — stay calm and avoid walking or driving.
2. **Chew one regular (325 mg) or four baby (81 mg) aspirins** *(ask 911) only if your provider has told you it's safe and you have no allergy or bleeding issues.*
3. **Unlock your door** so help can reach you quickly.
4. **Have medication lists and emergency contacts ready.**

Emergency Room

- Bring your medication list and insurance card to the ER.
- Write down what the hospital team tells you — or have someone take notes.
- Ask when to follow up with your cardiologist or provider.

Remember: Fast action saves heart muscle — and lives.

See the back for a tear out condensed version of this to keep near your phone or taped inside your medication cabinet.

Table of Contents

SECTION 1

Understanding Your Heart

Your Body's Powerhouse Pump

Introduction

Heart disease is one of the most common health problems in the world — but it's also one of the most **treatable and preventable**.

Heart disease is a broad term that includes many problems like blocked arteries, heart attacks, or valve disease. Heart failure is one kind of heart disease — it happens when the heart becomes weak or stiff over time.

The truth is, understanding how the heart works and what puts it at risk can help you make better choices, get help sooner, and live a longer, healthier life.

You don't need to be a medical expert to take good care of your heart. This book is written in **plain language** to help you understand what's happening inside your body, what your medical provider may recommend, and what you can do every day to protect your heart.

Heart failure means your heart is weaker or stiffer than it used to be, so it can't pump blood as easily. It does *not* mean your heart has stopped.

Heart failure sounds frightening, but most people live for years with the right plan.

In this book, you'll find:

- What heart failure means
- What tests and treatments you may have
- What to do every day to stay well
- When to call for help

What This Book Will Teach You

Inside these pages, you'll learn:

- What your heart does and how it keeps your body alive
- What happens when the heart or blood vessels become diseased or blocked
- What is heart failure and why does it lead to big issues?
- The tests your provider may order and what they show
- The treatments — from medicines to surgeries — that can help your heart work better.
- How to care for yourself at home and what to expect in cardiac rehab
- How lifestyle changes, good nutrition, and exercise protect your heart
- What to do if you or someone you love has a heart emergency

Each chapter breaks complex ideas into easy steps and real examples, so you can follow along without medical training.

About the Patient Voice in This Book

- *Throughout this book, you'll hear from **Trish**, a patient currently living with **heart failure**.*
- *Her experiences bring the medical information in these pages to life – showing what it's really like to notice the first symptoms, go through testing, start new medications, and adjust to daily changes.*
- *Trish's reflections appear throughout the chapters to remind readers that heart disease is more than numbers and test results – it's a lived experience that affects your body, emotions, and family.*
- *Her honesty and humor help make complex topics feel real and relatable. I am deeply grateful to Trish for sharing her journey so openly. Her voice represents the strength, vulnerability, and courage found in so many people facing heart disease.*

How common is Heart Failure?

- Approximately **6.7 million adults age 20 or older in the United States** have been diagnosed with heart failure. https://www.cdc.gov/heart-disease/about/heart-failure
- That number corresponds roughly to **1.9 % to 2.6 %** of U.S. adults overall.
- Lifetime risk: For an individual in the U.S., the lifetime risk of developing heart failure is estimated at about **1 in 4 (≈ 25 %)**. https://hfsa.org/heart-failure-hf-rate-expected-rise-85-million-americans-2030-new-hfsa-initiative-identifies
- This number is expected to **rise**: e.g., projected to reach ~8.5 million by 2030.
- Importantly: another statistic notes that **≈ 1/3 of U.S. adults** are at risk (Stage A) and 24-34 % may be in a "pre-heart failure" (Stage B) category, says the Heart Failure Society of America.

Why Understanding Helps You Feel Less Scared

When you understand your condition, you can notice warning signs sooner. You'll also be able to ask clearer questions and follow your plan with confidence. Understanding your condition also helps you:

- Ask better questions during appointments
- Notice warning signs early
- Manage medications safely
- Follow your care plan with confidence

Patient Perspective:
"I just thought I was getting asthma. My father had it, my sister had it, so I figured that's what it was. I started getting short of breath on walks, but I didn't think much of it. I just blamed being out of shape... I thought I was just getting older. I never dreamed it was my heart."

Remember: **knowledge is power, and preparation brings peace of mind.**

Trusted Information

The information in this book comes from:

- American College of Cardiology (ACC)
- Duke University Hospital
- Johns Hopkins Medicine
- Mayo Clinic
- Cleveland Clinic
- American Heart Association (AHA)
- Heart Failure Society of America

Every treatment or procedure described here is based on current medical guidelines used by heart specialists across the United States.

A Final Word Before You Begin

- Heart disease can be serious, but it is **not hopeless.**
- With the right care, many people live long, active, and meaningful lives.
- Your job is to learn, ask questions, and take small, steady steps toward heart health — one day at a time.
- Whether you're reading this for yourself, a loved one, or a patient you care for, this book is your partner in understanding and confidence.
- Let's start by learning how your heart works — and how you can protect it for years to come.
- Your kidneys and heart work together—when one struggles, the other feels it

Heart Disease at a Glance

Your heart is about the size of your fist — small enough to fit in your hand, but powerful enough to move blood through thousands of miles of blood vessels every single day. It never rests for long. Even when you're asleep, it keeps pumping, sending oxygen and nutrients to every organ and cell in your body.

How the Heart Works

Think of your heart like a **two-story house with four rooms and some very smart plumbing.**

- The **right side** of the house handles "used" blood that has already delivered oxygen to the body.
- The **left side** handles "fresh" blood coming back from the lungs, filled with oxygen and ready to go out again.
- The **walls and doors** between the rooms keep blood flowing in the right direction and make sure nothing leaks backward.
- The **pipes** are your arteries and veins, carrying blood to and from the heart.

Each heartbeat is like the plumbing system turning on — filling, pumping, and sending blood where it needs to go.

The Heart's Electrical System

Your heart is both a **pump** and an **electrical system** — like an engine with spark plugs and pistons working together.

The Four Chambers

Your heart's four "rooms":

- **Right Atrium:** collects blood returning from your body that's low in oxygen.
- **Right Ventricle:** sends that blood to your lungs to pick up oxygen.
- **Left Atrium:** receives the oxygen-rich blood coming back from the lungs.

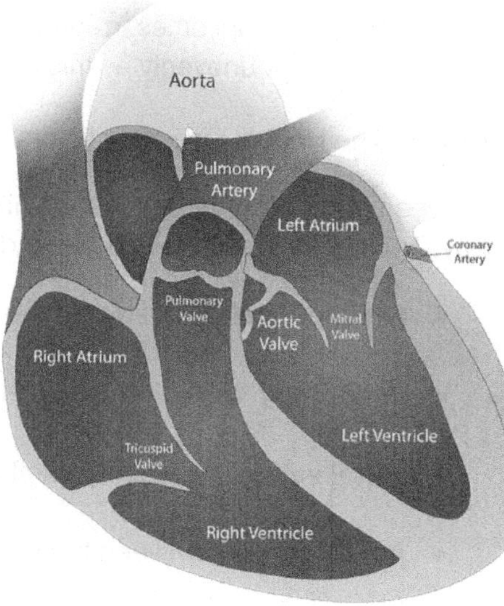

- **Left Ventricle:** pumps that oxygen-rich blood through the aorta to your whole body.
- The **left ventricle** is the strongest room — it does most of the heavy work.
- **Ejection Fraction** is the percentage of blood your heart pumps out each beat. A normal ejection fraction (EF) is about 50–70 %. Think of it as your heart's 'score' for how well it pumps.

The Electrical Wiring

- Every heartbeat begins with a tiny electrical signal in the **SA node**, your heart's natural pacemaker.
- That signal travels through the **AV node** and down into the lower chambers, telling them when to squeeze.
- This happens about **60–100 times per minute** — that's your pulse.
- If the wiring becomes irregular, the heart may beat too fast, too slow, or unevenly — this is called an **arrhythmia.**

Valves: The Heart's One-Way Doors

Between each chamber are **valves**, like doors that only open one way. They keep blood moving forward.

- **Tricuspid valve** – between the right atrium and right ventricle
- **Pulmonary valve** – between the right ventricle and the lungs
- **Mitral valve** – between the left atrium and left ventricle
- **Aortic valve** – between the left ventricle and the aorta

If a valve doesn't open or close properly, it can cause murmurs, leaks, or pressure problems (you'll learn more in the valve chapter later).

Arteries and Veins: The Highway System

Your blood vessels are like a giant **road network.**

- **Arteries** carry blood *away* from the heart. They're the highways that deliver oxygen-rich blood to your muscles and organs.
- **Veins** bring blood *back* to the heart after the oxygen has been used.
- The **aorta** is the main highway leaving the heart — it branches out into smaller roads (arteries) that reach every part of the body.
- The **vena cava** is the main road bringing blood back home.

The **Lungs** and the "Round Trip"

Every drop of blood takes a full round trip:

1. From the body → to the right side of the heart → to the lungs

2. From the lungs → to the left side of the heart → back out to the body

That trip happens about **once every second.**

Blood Pressure: The Push Behind the Flow

When your heart squeezes, it creates pressure to push blood through your vessels.

This is called **blood pressure**, and it's written as two numbers — like 120/80.

- The top number (**systolic**) is the push when the heart squeezes.

- The bottom number (**diastolic**) is the pressure when it relaxes and refills.

Healthy blood pressure keeps your arteries strong and reduces stress on your heart.

How It All Works Together

Think of the heart, blood, and lungs as a **team:**

- The **heart** pumps the blood.
- The **lungs** fill it with oxygen.
- The **arteries and veins** deliver and return it.
- Your heart also has its own built-in electrical system that tells it when to beat.
- Problems with this system can cause irregular rhythms called arrhythmias. These are the SA node and AV node, see arrhythmia section for more details.
- When all three work together, your cells get what they need to stay alive and full of energy.
- When one part struggles — like a clogged artery or weak muscle — the whole system feels the effect.

What You Can Do Right Now

- *Learn your normal blood pressure and pulse.*
- *Notice your body's signals — shortness of breath, swelling, or chest discomfort.*
- *Ask your provider to explain your test results in simple words.*
- *Keep this book nearby as a reference when you hear medical terms.*

Patient Perspective: "When my cardiologist first showed me a picture of my heart, I thought — that can't be me! Seeing how the chambers and valves actually work helped me understand why every pill and every ounce of water matters."

✎ **Notes:**

What new things did I learn about how my heart works?

What questions should I ask my provider about my heart anatomy or function?

Key Terms for this Section

Atrium (AY-tree-um):
The upper chambers of the heart that collect blood coming in. There's a right atrium and a left atrium.

Ventricle (VEN-trih-kul):
The lower chambers that pump blood out of the heart.

Valve:
A one-way "door" that keeps blood moving in the right direction.

Aorta (ay-OR-tuh):
The largest artery that carries oxygen-rich blood from the heart to the rest of the body.

Pulmonary (PULL-muh-nair-ee):
Means "related to the lungs." The pulmonary artery and vein connect the heart and lungs.

Artery:
A blood vessel that carries blood *away* from the heart.

Vein:
A blood vessel that carries blood *back* to the heart.

SA Node (Sinoatrial Node):
The heart's natural "spark plug" that starts each heartbeat.

Blood Pressure:
The force of blood pushing against your arteries when the heart squeezes and relaxes.

Pulse:
The rhythmic beat you feel when the heart pumps blood through your body.

SECTION 2

Preparing for First Office Visit

What to think about before you go

Preparing for your first Cardiology Visit

- Going to see a cardiologist (heart specialist) for the first time can feel overwhelming.
- You might be worried they'll find something serious — or that you won't understand the medical words they use.
- But here's the truth: the goal of your visit isn't to scare you — it's to **find answers, create a plan, and protect your heart for the long run.**
- The more prepared you are, the easier the visit will feel.
- Think of it like getting ready for a trip — you want to bring the right information and know what questions to ask once you get there.

Patient Perspective: "Don't wait like I did. If you're short of breath or your legs feel heavy, pay attention. I used to think I was bothering my doctors – not anymore. If I have symptoms now, they know about it. Some people don't want to know because they're afraid of bad news. But waiting doesn't fix anything. The earlier you catch it, the better your life will be."

What to Bring

Your medical provider can help you best when they have the full picture.

Before your visit, gather and bring:

- ☐ A **list of your current medications**, including vitamins and over-the-counter drugs
- ☐ **Names and contact information** for your other medical providers
- ☐ **Recent test results** or hospital records, if available
- ☐ **Blood pressure or weight logs**, if you've been tracking at home
- ☐ A **list of your symptoms** — when they started, what they feel like, and what makes them better or worse
- ☐ Your **insurance card** and photo ID

Here are the 12 Most Common Symptoms of Heart Failure
(Source: American Heart Association, 2022 ACC/AHA/HFSA Heart Failure Guidelines.)

1. **Shortness of Breath (Dyspnea):** Feeling winded during everyday activities, like climbing stairs or walking short distances, is one of the earliest and most common signs of heart failure.

   It may also happen when lying flat (orthopnea) or waking suddenly at night gasping for air (paroxysmal nocturnal dyspnea).

2. **Fatigue or Weakness:** The heart's reduced pumping ability means less oxygen reaches your muscles. You might notice you tire easily, can't walk as far as before, or feel drained doing routine tasks.

3. **Swelling (Edema) and Fluid Retention:** When blood backs up, fluid can collect in the legs, ankles, feet, or belly. Shoes may feel tighter, or you may notice unexplained weight gain of a few pounds in just days.

4. **Persistent Cough or Wheezing:** Fluid buildup in the lungs can cause a long-lasting cough or wheeze, especially when lying down or at night.

   This may sound like asthma but is actually a sign of heart congestion.

5. **Rapid or Irregular Heartbeat (Palpitations):** As the heart struggles to pump efficiently, it may beat faster or with skipped beats.

   You might feel fluttering, pounding, or a racing sensation in your chest.

6. **Loss of Appetite or Nausea:** When the liver and stomach get congested with fluid, you may feel full quickly, lose interest in food, or feel bloated or nauseated after small meals.

7. **Frequent Nighttime Urination (Nocturia):** Fluid that gathers in your legs during the day can return to the bloodstream when lying down, causing increased urination at night.

8. **Abdominal Swelling or Sudden Weight Gain:** Beyond ankle swelling, heart failure can cause fluid to collect in the belly or back.

   A sudden increase of 2–3 pounds in 24 hours or 5 pounds in a week often signals fluid retention.

9. **Lightheadedness, Dizziness, or Confusion:** Reduced blood flow to the brain can make you feel dizzy, forgetful, or "foggy." These changes often appear subtly and may worsen when standing up. *Source: National Center for Biotechnology Information (NCBI), 2022.*

10. **Shortness of Breath at Rest or Minimal Activity:** As heart failure progresses, you may feel winded even while talking, dressing, or resting quietly. This can indicate worsening fluid buildup in the lungs. *Source: PMC Heart Failure Review, 2023.*

11. **Neck Vein Swelling (Jugular Venous Distention):** Your medical provider might notice bulging neck veins—a sign of fluid buildup and pressure in the venous system.

    While not a symptom you'll feel, it's an important exam finding.

12. **Reduced Exercise Tolerance:** You may no longer be able to do activities you once enjoyed—like gardening, walking the dog, or shopping—without feeling wiped out.

    This gradual decline is a key indicator that the heart isn't keeping up. *Source: ACC/AHA/HFSA 2022 Guidelines.*

Less Common Causes of Heart Failure

-Some heart problems are caused by genetic or infiltrative conditions such as amyloidosis, sarcoidosis, or iron overload.
-If several family members have heart issues or you developed symptoms young, ask about genetic or specialized testing.

Some Reversible Causes: Sometimes heart failure worsens because of other treatable conditions. Check that your provider is following these issues regularly:

- ☐ Low iron or anemia
- ☐ Thyroid problems
- ☐ Kidney changes
- ☐ Sleep apnea

Correcting these can improve energy, breathing, and quality of life.

What Your Provider Will Ask

Your cardiologist or advanced practice provider (PA, NP) will ask about your story — also known as your **HPI (History of Present Illness).** They'll want to understand what brought you in and what you've been feeling.

Here are some common questions to think about ahead of time:

Symptoms and Changes

When did you first notice shortness of breath, swelling, or fatigue?

Are your symptoms getting better, worse, or about the same?

Do you ever wake up at night short of breath or need extra pillows to sleep?

Have you noticed swelling in your feet, ankles, legs, or belly?

Do you ever feel your heart racing, skipping beats, or pounding in your chest?

Have you gained or lost weight unexpectedly in the past few days or weeks?

Do you ever feel dizzy, lightheaded, or more forgetful than usual?

Notes:

Activity and Daily Living

How far can you walk or climb stairs before feeling short of breath or tired?

Have you had to stop doing any usual activities (like gardening, walking, shopping)?

How many pillows do you sleep with at night, and can you lie flat comfortably?

Are you still able to do your usual chores, or do you need help?

Notes:

Diet and Fluid Intake

How much fluid do you drink in a day? (Your provider may give you a limit.)

Do you use salt when cooking or at the table?

Have you noticed any bloating or loss of appetite?

Notes:

Medications

Are you taking your heart medications exactly as prescribed?

Have you missed any doses recently or run out of medication?

Do you know the names of your medicines and what they're for?

Have you noticed any side effects, such as dizziness, cough, or swelling?

Notes:

Weight and Monitoring

Do you weigh yourself every morning?

What was your most recent weight change?

Do you keep a record or use a daily tracker?

Notes:

Patient Perspective: "They told me to weigh myself every morning. If I gain two pounds in two days, I have to call the doctor. I lost six pounds of water in the hospital – that's when I realized how much fluid I'd been carrying."

Other Medical History

Have you ever been told you had a heart attack or heart valve problem?

Do you have high blood pressure, diabetes, or kidney problems?

Have you had any recent hospital stays or ER visits for your heart?

Is there any family history of heart problems or heart failure?

Notes:

Patient Perspective: "My mother had heart failure. So did my grandmother. Now my sister's been diagnosed too...It runs in the family, but I didn't think it would happen to me – until it did."

Lifestyle and Support

Do you smoke, vape, or drink alcohol?

How is your sleep, mood, or stress level lately?

Do you live alone or have help at home if you need it?

Do you feel safe and able to manage your medications, meals, and doctor visits?

Notes:

End-of-Life and Long-Term Planning (if applicable)

Have you discussed your wishes about advanced care (DNR/DNI, living will)?

Do you have someone who could make healthcare decisions for you if you couldn't?

Notes:

Questions You or Your Person May Want to Ask Your Provider:

- Being diagnosed with heart failure can feel overwhelming, and it's normal to have questions.
- Bringing this list to your visit can help you start an open, honest conversation with your cardiologist or advanced practice provider (PA or NP).
- You don't need to ask every question — just the ones that matter most to you right now.

Understanding Your Diagnosis

What type of heart failure do I have — is my heart too weak, too stiff, or both?

What stage or class of heart failure am I in?

How serious is my condition right now?

Can my heart function improve, or will it likely stay the same?

Is this considered a lifelong condition, or can it get better with treatment?

Treatment and Prognosis

Can my heart failure be managed with medications alone?

What are the main goals of my treatment plan?

How will we know if the medications are working?

Are there any procedures or surgeries that might help my heart work better?

What can I expect over the next few months or years?

Is heart failure something people die from, or can it be controlled long-term?

Notes:

Lifestyle and Daily Living

What changes should I make to my diet, fluids, or salt intake?

Is it safe for me to exercise, and what kind of activity do you recommend?

Will I need to check my blood pressure, weight, or oxygen at home?

Do you think I'll need special medical equipment (like oxygen or a home scale)?

Are there warning signs that mean I should call your office or go to the ER right away?

Notes:

Support and Planning

How often will I need follow-up visits or testing?

Should I see a heart failure specialist or join a cardiac rehab program?

Are there support groups or educational programs for people with heart failure?

Should I talk with a social worker about home care, medication costs, or transportation?

When is the right time to talk about advance directives (DNR/DNI or living will)?

Patient perspective: "I write my questions down on paper before every visit. Otherwise, I forget half of what I meant to ask. The doctors don't mind — they actually like that I come prepared."

Notes:

Tips for a Great Appointment

- ☐ Arrive early to fill out paperwork.
- ☐ Bring a support person if possible — they can help take notes or remember details.
- ☐ Write things down as you go.
- ☐ Be honest about your habits and symptoms — your provider can only help with what they know.
- ☐ Ask for a printed copy of your after-visit summary.
- ☐ You can even bring this book along to jot down new terms or advice during your visit.

After Your Appointment

Once you get home:

- ☐ Review your notes while the visit is still fresh.
- ☐ Write down any new medications or lifestyle recommendations.
- ☐ Schedule any follow-up tests right away so you don't forget.
- ☐ Share what you learned with your family — having support helps you stay on track.

Key Terms from This Section

Cardiologist:
A doctor who specializes in diagnosing and treating heart problems.

HPI (History of Present Illness):
The story you tell your provider about your symptoms — when they started and how they feel.

Family History:
Medical conditions that run in your family and may increase your risk.

After-Visit Summary:
A written report you get after your appointment listing your tests, medications, and next steps.

SECTION 3

Women and Heart Failure

How things are different

Unique Risks and Considerations

- Heart failure doesn't affect everyone the same way.
- Women often experience different symptoms, causes, and challenges than men.
- Understanding these differences can help women recognize changes sooner and take control of their heart health.

How Symptoms May Differ for Women

Women with heart failure often describe their symptoms differently. Instead of sharp chest pain, they may notice:

- Feeling more **tired or short of breath** than usual
- Swelling in the **legs, ankles, or belly**
- Needing **extra pillows to sleep** or waking up short of breath
- Feeling "foggy," anxious, or emotional for no clear reason

Because these signs can be subtle, they're sometimes mistaken for stress, menopause, or aging. Listening to your body and mentioning small changes to your provider can make a big difference.

Hormonal and Age-Related Factors

- Before menopause, estrogen helps protect a woman's heart by keeping blood vessels flexible and blood pressure stable.
- After menopause, lower estrogen levels can cause the heart muscle and arteries to become **stiffer**, making it harder for the heart to fill and pump efficiently.
- This is one reason why older women are more likely than men to develop **heart failure with preserved ejection fraction (HFpEF)** — sometimes called the "stiff heart" type.
- Maintaining good blood pressure control, staying active, and limiting salt can help prevent these changes over time.

Patient perspective: "After menopause, I blamed everything on getting older — the fatigue, the swelling, the shortness of breath. I wish I'd known those were heart symptoms, not just age catching up with me."

Pregnancy-Related Heart Risks

Pregnancy places extra stress on the heart, and certain complications can increase a woman's long-term risk of heart failure. These include:

- **Preeclampsia** (high blood pressure during pregnancy)
- **Gestational hypertension**
- **Gestational diabetes**
- **Peripartum cardiomyopathy** — a rare but serious form of heart failure that can develop in the last month of pregnancy or within months after delivery

Women who've had these conditions should tell their medical provider, even years later. Heart health checkups, blood pressure control, and healthy weight management can help reduce the risk of later heart problems.

Emotional and Lifestyle Differences

- Women often juggle caregiving roles, jobs, and family responsibilities — all while managing their own health.
- This constant stress can make it harder to follow a heart failure care plan or notice early warning signs.
- Women are also more likely to experience **anxiety or depression** after a diagnosis, which can affect energy, appetite, and medication routines.
- Building a support network, joining a cardiac rehab program, and talking openly about emotional health can all improve long-term outcomes.

Family Screening and Prevention

- Heart failure can sometimes run in families, especially if relatives have high blood pressure, diabetes, obesity, or inherited heart muscle conditions.
- Encourage family members to get regular blood pressure and cholesterol checks — even if they feel healthy.
- Simple steps like staying active, eating a balanced diet, and keeping a healthy weight can lower the risk for everyone in the family.

Knowing these signs early could save you from a hospital stay.

Key Takeaway

- Heart failure in women often starts with small, easily overlooked symptoms — not dramatic ones.
- By recognizing these early signs, staying on top of routine care, and sharing family and pregnancy history with your provider, women can protect their hearts and live active, fulfilling lives.

References

American College of Cardiology (ACC), American Heart Association (AHA), Heart Failure Society of America (HFSA) 2022–2024 Guidelines for the Management of Heart Failure; *Circulation* (2023); *Journal of the American College of Cardiology* (2022–2024); *UpToDate*, reviewed 2025; *National Institutes of Health (NIH) Office of Research on Women's Health*; *Centers for Disease Control and Prevention (CDC), Heart Disease and Women.*

Key Terms for This Section

Estrogen:
A hormone that helps protect blood vessels and cholesterol balance in women before menopause.

Family History:
Heart problems in close relatives (parents, siblings, or children) that raise your own risk.

Gestational Diabetes:
High blood sugar that develops during pregnancy; raises long-term heart risk.

Heart Failure with Preserved Ejection Fraction (HFpEF):
A type of heart failure where the heart muscle becomes stiff and cannot fill properly, even though its pumping strength looks normal on tests. More common in older women.

Menopause:
The time when menstrual periods stop and hormone levels decrease, increasing heart risk.

Peripartum Cardiomyopathy:
Heart weakness that occurs during pregnancy or soon after birth.

Postmenopausal:
The period of life after menopause when estrogen levels remain low, increasing the risk for high blood pressure, heart stiffness, and heart failure.

Preeclampsia:
High blood pressure during pregnancy that can harm the heart, kidneys, and other organs.

Pregnancy-Related Heart Risk:
Conditions that develop during pregnancy—such as preeclampsia, gestational hypertension, or gestational diabetes—that raise a woman's chance of developing heart failure later in life.

Stress and Emotional Health:
Mental and emotional strain that can raise blood pressure, heart rate, and inflammation over time, affecting heart health and recovery.

SECTION 4

Men and Heart Failure

What Makes It Different

Unique Risks and Considerations

- Heart failure affects men and women in different ways.
- Men often develop heart problems earlier in life and for different reasons.
- Understanding these differences helps men recognize symptoms sooner and take steps to protect their heart health.

How Symptoms May Differ for Men

- Men with heart failure tend to experience more **classic, physical symptoms** early on — such as shortness of breath, swelling in the legs, or sudden weight gain.
- They are also more likely to have a **weaker pumping heart** (called *heart failure with reduced ejection fraction*, or **HFrEF**) caused by prior heart attacks or long-term high blood pressure.
- Because men may downplay early symptoms or push through fatigue, they sometimes delay getting checked until the condition worsens.
- Talking with a provider as soon as symptoms appear can help prevent serious complications.

Knowing these signs early could save you from a hospital stay.

Notes:

Hormonal and Age-Related Factors

- Testosterone and other male hormones influence how the heart muscle repairs itself after injury.
- As men age and testosterone levels drop, the heart muscle can become **weaker or scarred**, especially after a heart attack.
- Men also tend to develop **artery plaque buildup (coronary artery disease)** earlier than women, increasing their risk for heart failure at a younger age.
- Regular check-ups for blood pressure, cholesterol, and diabetes are key to catching problems early — long before the heart begins to fail.

Lifestyle and Occupational Factors

- Men are more likely to have jobs or hobbies that involve **physical strain, long hours, or high stress**, all of which can raise blood pressure and heart rate over time.
- They may also be more likely to smoke, drink alcohol, or avoid medical visits until symptoms interfere with daily life.
- Small, steady lifestyle changes — quitting smoking, limiting alcohol, managing stress, and staying active — can lower heart failure risk and help treatment work better once diagnosed.

Notes:

Patient perspective: "My brother didn't go to the doctor until he couldn't walk from the car to the house without stopping. Men like to tough it out, but sometimes that toughness makes things worse."

Emotional Health and Social Support

- Men sometimes find it harder to talk about feelings like fear, frustration, or depression after being diagnosed with heart failure.
- Ignoring these emotions can make it harder to follow treatment plans or notice changes in symptoms.
- Building a support system — whether that's a partner, friend, or cardiac rehab group — can improve both mood and long-term outcomes.

Family History and Prevention

- Men are more likely to have **early-onset heart disease** in their families.
- If your father, brother, or son was diagnosed with heart failure or had a heart attack before age 55, your own risk is higher.
- Encourage male relatives to know their blood pressure, cholesterol, and weight — and to have regular heart screenings.
- Prevention is most effective when it starts early.

Key Takeaway

- Men often develop heart failure earlier in life, usually from artery disease or long-term high blood pressure.
- Paying attention to early symptoms, managing lifestyle risks, and staying consistent with medical care can make a major difference in how well and how long the heart functions.

Notes:

References

American College of Cardiology (ACC), American Heart Association (AHA), and Heart Failure Society of America (HFSA) Guidelines for the Management of Heart Failure 2022–2024; *Journal of the American College of Cardiology* (2022–2024); *Circulation* (2023); *UpToDate*, reviewed 2025; *Centers for Disease Control and Prevention (CDC), Heart Disease and Men.*

Key Terms for This Section

Alcohol Use:
Drinking too much alcohol over time can weaken the heart muscle and raise blood pressure, leading to heart failure.

Artery Disease (Coronary Artery Disease or CAD):
A buildup of plaque inside the arteries that supply blood to the heart. This reduces blood flow and can cause heart attacks, a leading cause of heart failure in men.

Blood Pressure (Hypertension):
The force of blood pushing against the walls of your arteries. When it stays high for years, it can enlarge or weaken the heart.

Cholesterol:
A waxy, fat-like substance in the blood. Too much "bad" cholesterol (LDL) can cause plaque buildup and blockages in the arteries.

Depression:
A mood disorder that can make it harder to follow medical instructions or stay motivated. Common in men with heart failure but often overlooked.

Ejection Fraction (EF):
The percentage of blood pumped out of the left ventricle with each heartbeat. A normal EF is usually between 50 – 70 %.

Heart Failure with Reduced Ejection Fraction (HFrEF):
A type of heart failure where the heart muscle is weakened and can't pump enough blood to meet the body's needs. More

common in men.

High-Stress Lifestyle:
A pattern of long work hours, poor sleep, or constant tension that increases heart rate, blood pressure, and inflammation over time.

Occupational Risk:
Job-related factors (physical labor, shift work, exposure to chemicals, or high stress) that may raise the risk of heart disease or heart failure.

Smoking:
Inhaling tobacco damages blood vessels, lowers oxygen in the blood, and greatly increases the risk of heart attack and heart failure.

Testosterone:
The main male hormone that supports muscle strength and heart function. Levels drop with age, which may affect how the heart repairs itself after injury.

Weight Management:
Maintaining a healthy body weight helps control blood pressure and reduces strain on the heart muscle.

SECTION 5

Understanding Heart Failure

Causes, Types, and Treatments

Let's Learn More

This section explains what causes heart failure and how your medical provider decides which treatment is best for you.

- Heart failure doesn't happen overnight.
- It develops slowly as the heart muscle weakens, stiffens, or becomes overloaded with pressure or fluid.
- Understanding the type and cause of your heart failure helps guide the right treatment plan for you.

Heart Failure Types:
There are three main patterns doctors use to describe heart function:

HFrEF=Heart failure with reduced Ejection Fraction	The heart muscle is weak and doesn't pump out enough blood
HFmrEF=Heart failure with midrange Ejection Fraction	The pumping strength is mildly reduced
HFpEF=Heart failure with preserved Ejection Fraction	The pumping strength looks normal, but the heart is stiff and doesn't fill easily

Notes:

Heart Failure Stages (A–D)
Heart failure is often described by *stage* and *class* — this helps providers match treatments to your needs.

- **Stage A:** At risk for heart failure but no heart damage yet (for example: high blood pressure, diabetes, obesity, or family history).
- **Stage B:** Heart changes are seen on testing, but you don't have symptoms yet.
- **Stage C:** You have symptoms like fatigue, swelling, or shortness of breath with activity.
- **Stage D:** Symptoms continue even at rest or you've needed hospital or advanced device therapy.

NYHA Classes (I–IV) describe how much activity causes symptoms:

- **Class I:** No symptoms with usual activity
- **Class II:** Mild symptoms with regular activity
- **Class III:** Symptoms with light activity
- **Class IV:** Symptoms even at rest

What is Cardiomyopathy (Heart Muscle Problems)

Cardiomyopathy means that the heart muscle itself has become damaged or changed in a way that makes it harder for the heart to pump blood.

It doesn't happen overnight — over time, the muscle may become **too weak, too thick, or too stiff.**

Depending on the cause, this can lead to symptoms like tiredness, swelling, shortness of breath, or irregular heartbeat. The word **cardiomyopathy** means "disease of the heart muscle." There are several types, each with different causes:

- **Dilated Cardiomyopathy:** The heart muscle becomes stretched and thin, making it harder to pump blood.

Common causes: past heart attacks, long-term high blood pressure, alcohol overuse, certain infections, or genetics.

- **Hypertrophic Cardiomyopathy:** The heart muscle (especially the left ventricle) becomes abnormally thick, leaving less room for blood to fill.

This can be inherited and may cause shortness of breath, chest pain, or fainting.

- **Restrictive Cardiomyopathy:** The heart walls become stiff but not thickened, so the heart can't relax and fill properly.

This may happen from conditions like amyloidosis or after radiation or chemotherapy.

- **Ischemic Cardiomyopathy:** Long-term reduced blood flow from blocked arteries weakens parts of the heart muscle–This is the *most common* cause of heart failure in men.

- **Peripartum Cardiomyopathy:** A rare type that develops during the last month of pregnancy or within several months after delivery.

Sometimes, heart failure isn't caused by a weak or stiff heart muscle — it's caused by a problem with the **heart's valves**, the one-way doors that control blood flow.

When a valve doesn't open all the way or doesn't close tightly, the heart has to work much harder to keep blood moving forward.

Over time, this extra strain can weaken the heart muscle and lead to heart failure.

The Role of Heart Valves

The heart has **four valves** that open and close to keep blood moving in the right direction:

1. **Aortic Valve** — between the left ventricle and the aorta
2. **Mitral Valve** — between the left atrium and left ventricle
3. **Tricuspid Valve** — between the right atrium and right ventricle
4. **Pulmonic Valve** — between the right ventricle and pulmonary artery

When these valves don't open or close properly, the heart must work harder, leading to heart failure over time.

- **Stenosis:** The valve is narrowed and doesn't open fully.
- **Regurgitation (Leak):** The valve doesn't close tightly, allowing blood to flow backward.

Valve disease can often be repaired or replaced through minimally invasive or surgical procedures, which can greatly improve heart function.

- Most cases of heart failure develop **slowly** over time, but sometimes symptoms can appear suddenly.
- When the heart is placed under extra stress — from a heart attack, infection, medication change, or sudden rise in blood pressure — it can struggle to keep up.
- This **sudden** worsening is called acute heart failure, and it often needs quick medical attention to remove extra fluid and stabilize breathing.

Acute (Sudden) Heart Failure

- Sometimes heart failure symptoms appear suddenly — this is called **acute heart failure**.
- It can happen after a heart attack, infection, medication change, or severe high blood pressure episode.
- Patients may feel short of breath, dizzy, or notice rapid weight gain and swelling.
- This usually requires hospital care, IV medicines, or oxygen therapy to remove fluid and stabilize breathing.

Patient perspective: "My first hospital stay scared me to death. I thought it meant the end. But it was actually the start of finally feeling better — they got the fluid off, changed my meds, and I could breathe again."

Notes:

Medical Treatments and Medications

Most people with heart failure take several medications that work together to help the heart pump more efficiently and reduce strain.

"The Big Four" = Core Medicines for Most Patients
These are the foundation of modern heart-failure treatment:

ARNI=angiotensin receptor-neprilysin inhibitor	Relaxes blood vessels and lowers stress hormones to the heart
Beta-blocker	Slows heart rate, improves pumping, and reduces hospitalizations.
Aldosterone blocker	Helps remove salt and water while protecting the heart muscle
SGLT2 inhibitor	Helps the heart and kidneys work together and reduces flare-ups

These medicines work best when used together and slowly increased to full dose under your provider's guidance.

Some basic information about medications:

Diuretics ("Water Pills")

- Reduce extra fluid and swelling
- Examples: *Furosemide (Lasix®), Bumetanide (Bumex®), Torsemide (Demadex®)*
- **Important:** Weigh yourself daily — a sudden 2–3 lb gain may mean fluid buildup.

Diuretic Equivalents and Goal

40 mg furosemide ≈ 20 mg torsemide ≈ 1 mg bumetanide.

The goal is comfort and steady breathing — not a specific number on the scale.

Patient Perspective: "Those water pills are a nuisance. I plan my day around when I can take them. I take my diuretic when I get home – otherwise, I'd spend my whole time out looking for a bathroom. I take about 14 pills a day. We space them out so I can keep track—I need more diuretics, but they can't increase them because of my kidneys. My GFR went as low as 39, but it's back to 50 now – they're very careful with my fluid pills. It's all about balance. Too little and I swell up, too much and it's hard on my kidneys."

ACE Inhibitors and ARBs

- Relax blood vessels and lower blood pressure
- Reduce stress on the heart and prevent worsening of heart failure
- Examples: *Lisinopril, Enalapril, Losartan, Valsartan*

ARNI

- Combines two mechanisms into one medicine — the leading standard for many heart failure patients
- Example: *Sacubitril/valsartan (Entresto®)*

Beta-Blockers

- Slow the heart rate and allow the heart to fill more completely
- Help prevent arrhythmias and improve survival
- Examples: *Carvedilol, Metoprolol succinate, Bisoprolol*

Aldosterone Antagonists

- Help the body get rid of sodium and water while preserving potassium
- Examples: *Spironolactone, Eplerenone*

SGLT2 Inhibitors

- Originally used for diabetes but proven to help heart failure symptoms and hospitalizations
- Examples: *Dapagliflozin (Farxiga®), Empagliflozin (Jardiance®)*

Notes:

HFpEF Care ("Stiff Heart" Type)

For people with preserved ejection fraction, the goals are controlling blood pressure, maintaining a healthy weight, treating sleep apnea, managing atrial fibrillation, and using SGLT2 inhibitors when appropriate.

Vasodilators and Nitrates

- Relax blood vessels and improve blood flow; especially helpful in some patients who cannot tolerate ACE inhibitors
- Examples: *Hydralazine, Isosorbide dinitrate*

Anticoagulants (Blood Thinners)

- Used if you have atrial fibrillation or blood clots to prevent stroke
- Examples: *Apixaban (Eliquis®), Rivaroxaban (Xarelto®), Warfarin (Coumadin®)*

Other Helpful Treatments

- **IV Iron (for low iron):** Can improve energy and reduce hospital visits when ferritin is under 100 or between 100–300 with low transferrin saturation.

- **Weight Loss and GLP-1 Medicines:** For overweight patients with HFpEF, medications such as semaglutide (Wegovy®) can improve exercise tolerance and symptoms.

- **Sleep Apnea Treatment:** CPAP or BiPAP therapy helps reduce strain on the heart and improves oxygen levels.

Medicines to Avoid or Use Carefully (always discuss with your medical team)

- Avoid NSAIDs (ibuprofen, naproxen) — they cause fluid retention.
- Avoid cold medicines with pseudoephedrine — they raise blood pressure.
- Pause SGLT2 inhibitors and ACE/ARB/ARNI if you are vomiting, dehydrated, or have poor appetite until your provider advises to restart.

Patient Perspective: "I didn't know cold medicine could affect my heart until my provider caught it. Now I always check before taking anything new."

- Medications are often the first step — and for many people, they're enough to keep heart failure well controlled.
- But if symptoms continue despite the right medicines, your medical provider may discuss other treatment options that help the heart pump more effectively.
- These can include specialized devices or procedures designed to support or restore heart function.

Medical Devices and Procedures

In addition to medications, some patients benefit from specialized heart devices.

- **Implantable Cardioverter-Defibrillator (ICD):**
  Prevents sudden cardiac arrest by detecting and correcting dangerous rhythms.

- **Cardiac Resynchronization Therapy (CRT):**
  A pacemaker that helps the heart's chambers beat in sync for more efficient pumping.

- **Left Ventricular Assist Device (LVAD):**
  A mechanical pump used for severe heart failure when medications are no longer enough.

- **Valve Repair or Replacement:**
  Fixes leaking or narrowed valves that are worsening heart failure.

- **Heart Transplant:**
  Considered only when all other options have failed — rare but life-saving in select patients.

When to Ask About an ICD or CRT

If your ejection fraction is 35% or lower after 3 months of treatment and you still have symptoms, you may benefit from an implanted device:

- ICD helps prevent sudden cardiac arrest.

- CRT helps both sides of the heart beat in sync.
  Ask about this at your next follow-up echocardiogram.

- While devices like ICDs and CRTs are often used to help the heart pump more efficiently, they can also play an important role in managing heart rhythm problems.
- Heart rhythm issues, called arrhythmias, happen when the electrical system of the heart doesn't fire in the normal pattern.
- Some are harmless, but others can cause dizziness, shortness of breath, or even sudden cardiac arrest — which is why recognizing and treating them early is so important.

Understanding Heart Rhythm Problems (Arrhythmias)

Sometimes, heart failure causes the heart to beat too fast, too slow, or out of rhythm. These are called **arrhythmias**. They happen because damaged or stretched heart muscle can interrupt the heart's normal electrical signals.

- A **slow heartbeat (bradycardia)** can make you dizzy or tired.

- A **fast heartbeat (tachycardia)** can cause palpitations or shortness of breath.

- **Irregular rhythms** like *atrial fibrillation* (A-fib) can increase the risk of stroke.

Your provider may use medicines like **beta-blockers** or procedures like an **ICD** or **pacemaker** to help control these rhythms and keep your heart beating safely.

Notes:

Lifestyle and Self-Care

Daily habits make a major difference in how well you feel and how stable your heart failure stays.

- **Limit salt (sodium):** Aim for under 2,000 mg per day unless told otherwise.
- **Track your weight daily:** A gain of 2–3 lbs overnight may mean fluid buildup.
- **Take medicines consistently:** Never stop on your own — call your provider first.
- **Limit fluids** if recommended by your medical team.
- **Stay active** with light walking or cardiac rehab.
- **Avoid smoking and excess alcohol.**
- **Manage stress:** Mindfulness, breathing exercises, and counseling all help.
- **Keep follow-up visits:** Early adjustments prevent hospital stays.

Notes:

Key Takeaway

- Heart failure can often be controlled for many years with the right combination of medications, devices, and lifestyle changes.
- Knowing your type of cardiomyopathy, monitoring your symptoms, and staying consistent with treatment are the keys to living well.

References

American College of Cardiology (ACC), American Heart Association (AHA), Heart Failure Society of America (HFSA) *Guidelines for the Management of Heart Failure*, 2022–2024; *Journal of the American College of Cardiology* (2023); *Circulation* (2023); *UpToDate*, reviewed 2025.

Key Terms for this Section

ACE Inhibitor (Angiotensin-Converting Enzyme Inhibitor):
A medication that relaxes blood vessels and lowers blood pressure, reducing the heart's workload.

Acute Heart Failure:
A sudden worsening of heart failure symptoms such as shortness of breath, swelling, or fatigue that often requires hospital care.

Aldosterone Antagonist:
A medicine that helps remove extra fluid and sodium while keeping potassium in balance.

Aortic Valve:
The heart valve between the left ventricle and the aorta that controls blood flow out to the body.

ARNI (Angiotensin Receptor–Neprilysin Inhibitor):
A modern heart-failure medication that combines two actions—relaxing blood vessels and lowering stress hormones—to improve heart function (example: Entresto®).

Beta-Blocker:
A medication that slows the heart rate and lowers blood pressure so the heart can pump more efficiently.

Cardiac Resynchronization Therapy (CRT):
A special type of pacemaker that helps both sides of the heart beat together in rhythm.

Cardiomyopathy:
A disease of the heart muscle that makes it harder for the heart to pump blood.

Coronary Artery Disease (CAD):
Narrowing or blockage of the arteries that supply blood to the heart muscle; a leading cause of heart failure.

Diastolic Dysfunction / HFpEF (Heart Failure with Preserved Ejection Fraction):
A form of heart failure where the heart muscle is stiff and cannot relax or fill properly.

Diuretics ("Water Pills"):
Medications that help the body get rid of extra salt and water to reduce swelling and fluid buildup.

Ejection Fraction (EF):
The percentage of blood pumped out of the left ventricle with each heartbeat; a key measure of heart function.

Heart Valve:
One of four flaps (aortic, mitral, tricuspid, pulmonic) that open and close to keep blood flowing in the right direction.

HFrEF (Heart Failure with Reduced Ejection Fraction):
A type of heart failure where the heart muscle is weak and pumps out less blood than normal.

Hypertrophic Cardiomyopathy:
A thickened heart muscle that can limit blood flow and cause shortness of breath or fainting.

Implantable Cardioverter-Defibrillator (ICD):
A small device placed in the chest that shocks or paces the heart if a dangerous rhythm occurs.

Ischemic Cardiomyopathy:
Heart weakness caused by reduced blood flow or prior heart attacks that damage the muscle.

Left Ventricular Assist Device (LVAD):
A mechanical pump that helps the left side of the heart circulate blood when it is too weak to do so on its own.

Mitral Valve:
The valve between the left atrium and left ventricle; keeps blood moving forward into the ventricle.

Peripartum Cardiomyopathy:
A rare type of heart failure that develops during the last month of pregnancy or within months after delivery.

Pulmonic Valve:
The valve between the right ventricle and pulmonary artery that controls blood flow to the lungs.

Restrictive Cardiomyopathy:
A condition where the heart walls become stiff and can't fill with blood easily.

Right-Heart Catheterization:
A test that measures pressures inside the heart and lungs to guide fluid management and treatment.

SGLT2 Inhibitors:
A class of medicines originally for diabetes that also helps remove excess fluid and improve heart-failure outcomes (examples: Farxiga®, Jardiance®).

Stenosis:
A narrowing of a heart valve opening that makes the heart work harder to pump blood.

Tricuspid Valve:
The valve between the right atrium and right ventricle; helps control blood flow to the lungs.

Valve Regurgitation (Leak):
A valve problem where blood flows backward instead of moving forward through the heart.

SECTION 6

Testing and Diagnosis

What They are and What They Mean

When your provider suspects heart failure, several tests can help explain how well your heart is working and what may have caused the problem.

Some of these tests look at the *structure* of your heart, while others measure its *function* or the amount of stress it's under.

Blood Tests

Your heart releases a hormone called **B-type Natriuretic Peptide (BNP)** when it's stretched or working too hard.

A blood test can measure BNP or NT-proBNP to help confirm or rule out heart failure.

- **High levels** suggest your heart is struggling to pump effectively or that fluid is building up.
- **Lower or normal levels** make heart failure less likely.
- If you take certain medicines such as *Entresto (ARNI)*, your provider may order the **NT-proBNP** version because it's more accurate while on that drug.

These tests are also used to track progress — falling BNP levels often mean your treatment is working.

Notes:

More Testing

Electrocardiogram (EKG or ECG)

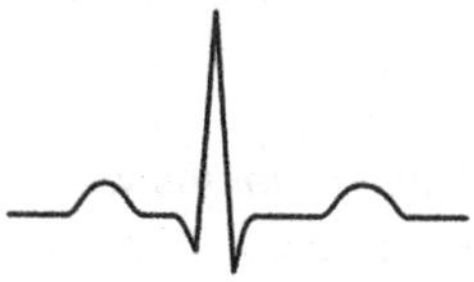

P–QRS–T = one heartbeat

- This quick test measures the heart's electrical signals through small stickers on your chest, arms, and legs.
- It can show rhythm problems, heart rate, past heart attacks, or patterns that suggest the heart muscle is enlarged or under strain.
- The machine records the pattern of electrical signals — like a graph showing your heart's rhythm.
- It only takes a few minutes and doesn't hurt.

Echocardiogram (Echo)

- An ultrasound of the heart that shows it in real time.
- It measures **ejection fraction (EF)** — the percentage of blood pumped out of the left ventricle with each beat.
- A **normal EF** is about 50–70%.
- A **low EF** means the heart is weak (*Heart Failure with Reduced Ejection Fraction — HFrEF*).

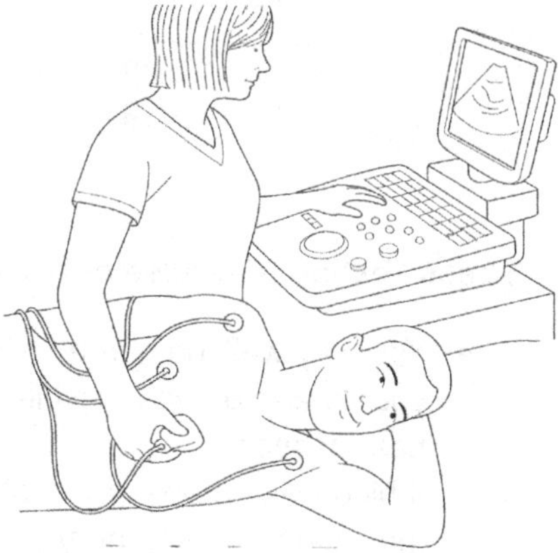

- A **normal EF but ongoing symptoms** suggests a *stiff heart* (*Heart Failure with Preserved Ejection Fraction — HFpEF*).

The echo also shows valve problems, wall motion, and overall heart size.

Patient perspective: "The echo felt strange — I could hear the whooshing of my own heartbeat. When the tech said my 'EF' was low, I had no clue what that meant until my provider explained it was my heart's 'score.'"

Chest X-Ray

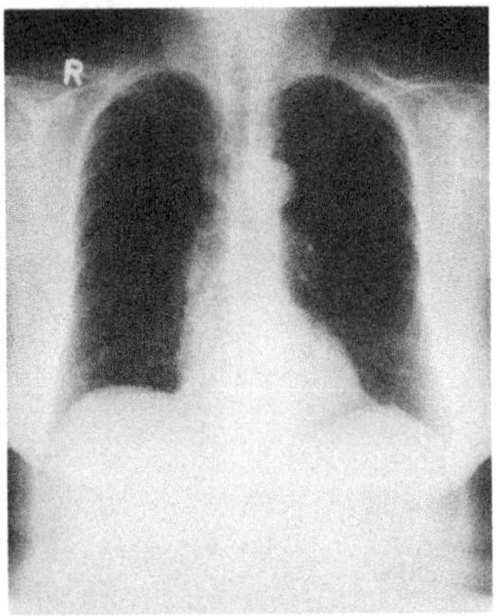

A simple picture of the heart and lungs that can reveal fluid buildup, lung congestion, or an enlarged heart shape — all common in heart failure.

Stress Testing (Exercise or Nuclear)

- You may walk on a treadmill or receive medicine that makes your heart beat faster while images or EKGs record how the heart responds.
- If blood flow drops or symptoms worsen during the test, it may mean blocked arteries are contributing to your heart failure.

CT Scan or CT Angiogram

- A CT angiogram uses contrast dye and detailed X-rays to check for blockages in coronary arteries.
- While this test mainly looks for *coronary artery disease*, identifying blockages helps explain *why* heart failure may have developed.

Calcium Scoring CT

- This scan measures calcium buildup in artery walls to estimate risk for future blockages.
- It's more useful for **heart-disease risk assessment** than for diagnosing heart failure, but your provider may recommend it if you have multiple risk factors.

Cardiac MRI

- An MRI creates highly detailed pictures of the heart muscle and surrounding tissues.
- It can detect **scarring, inflammation, or thickening** — helping identify specific causes like myocarditis, amyloidosis, or other cardiomyopathies.

Notes:

Cardiac Catheterization

During a cardiac catheterization, a long, thin tube called a catheter is gently placed into an artery — usually in your wrist or groin — and guided up toward your heart.

- A small amount of contrast dye is injected through the tube so that X-rays can show how well blood is flowing and if there are any narrow or blocked areas.
- A **left-heart cath** looks for blockages in the coronary arteries that may have caused the damage.
- A **right-heart cath** measures **pressures inside the heart and lungs**, helping guide treatment when fluid buildup or pulmonary hypertension is suspected.

You're awake but numbed, and most patients go home the same day.

Safety and Preparation Tips

- Wear comfortable clothing and remove jewelry.
- Don't eat or drink (except water) before tests that require fasting — your provider will tell you which ones.
- Bring a list of your medicines, allergies, and recent lab results.
- Tell your team if you're pregnant, have kidney disease, or have ever had a reaction to contrast dye.
- Most tests are painless, and recovery is usually quick.

Notes:

Understanding Your Results

Your medical team will review each test and explain what it means for your specific type of heart failure. Results help determine:

- How strong or stiff your heart muscle is
- Whether arteries or valves are contributing to the problem
- How much fluid or pressure is building up
- Which medications or procedures may help most

Keep a notebook or folder to track your test results, EF numbers, and BNP levels over time — it helps you and your care team see your progress clearly.

References

American College of Cardiology (ACC), American Heart Association (AHA), and Heart Failure Society of America (HFSA) Guidelines for the Management of Heart Failure (2022 – 2024); *Circulation* 2023; *Journal of the American College of Cardiology* 2022 – 2024; *UpToDate*, reviewed 2025.

What You Can Do Right Now

☐ *Keep copies of all your test reports or results.*

☐ *Write down what each test is for and when you had it.*

☐ *Ask your provider which tests you'll need regularly.*

Don't let fear stop you from getting tests — they're the best tools to protect your heart.

Key Terms

BNP (B-type Natriuretic Peptide):
A hormone released by the heart when it's stretched or under stress. High levels suggest heart failure or fluid buildup.

Calcium Scoring CT:
A special CT scan that measures calcium buildup in the coronary arteries to estimate future heart-disease risk.

Cardiac Catheterization (Heart Cath):
A procedure using thin tubes inserted through a blood vessel to measure heart pressures or look for blockages.

Cardiac MRI:
A magnetic-resonance imaging test that creates detailed pictures of the heart muscle, showing scarring, inflammation, or damage.

Chest X-ray:
A quick test that shows the size of the heart and whether there's fluid in the lungs.

Contrast Dye:
A liquid injected during some scans (like CT or MRI) to make blood vessels and heart structures easier to see.

CT Angiogram:
A CT scan that uses contrast dye to look for blockages in the heart's arteries.

Echocardiogram (Echo):
An ultrasound of the heart that measures pumping strength, valve function, and ejection fraction (EF).

Ejection Fraction (EF):
The percentage of blood the left ventricle pumps out with each heartbeat. A normal EF is about 50–70 percent.

Electrocardiogram (EKG or ECG):
A test that records the heart's electrical activity to find rhythm

problems, prior heart attacks, or strain on the heart.

HFrEF (Heart Failure with Reduced Ejection Fraction):
A type of heart failure where the heart muscle is weak and pumps out less blood than normal.

HFpEF (Heart Failure with Preserved Ejection Fraction):
A type of heart failure where the heart muscle is stiff and doesn't fill properly, even though pumping strength appears normal.

NT-proBNP:
A lab test similar to BNP, often used in people taking certain medications like Entresto®.

Nuclear Stress Test:
A test that uses a small amount of tracer dye to show blood flow to the heart during exercise or medication-induced stress.

Right-Heart Catheterization:
A cath procedure that measures pressures inside the heart and lungs to assess fluid overload or pulmonary hypertension.

Stress Test (Exercise Test):
A test that shows how the heart responds to activity. You may walk on a treadmill or take medication that mimics exercise.

SECTION 7

Cardiac Rehabilitation and Lifestyle Management

Recovering from heart failure is about more than just taking medicine.

How you move, eat, rest, and manage stress all affect how your heart performs day-to-day. The good news: many people with heart failure live full, active lives once they learn how to pace themselves and protect their hearts.

What Is Cardiac Rehabilitation?

Cardiac rehab is a medically supervised program designed for people recovering from heart problems such as heart failure, valve repair, or heart attack.

It usually includes:

- **Exercise training:** Gentle, safe workouts designed by specialists.
- **Education:** Learning how to read your symptoms, manage your medications, and make healthy choices.
- **Support:** Counseling, stress management, and connection with others living with heart disease.

Cardiac rehab helps rebuild strength, confidence, and independence — one step at a time.

Most programs meet two or three times per week for several weeks.

Ask your provider for a referral — it's covered by Medicare and most insurance plans.

Getting Active Safely

Physical activity keeps your heart and muscles strong, but it must be done **gradually and safely**.

Start with:

- **Short walks** (5–10 minutes) once or twice a day.
- Add a few minutes each week as tolerated.
- Rest when you need to — shortness of breath or fatigue that lasts more than a few minutes is a sign to slow down.

Avoid heavy lifting or straining until your provider clears you.

If you feel dizzy, have chest pressure, or can't catch your breath, stop and rest.

Everyday Activities: Stairs, Sex, Golf, and More

It's common to wonder when you can get back to your usual routines.

A simple rule of thumb: **if** you can walk two flights of stairs or briskly walk a block without symptoms, most daily activities — including sex — are generally safe.

But every patient is different, so **ask** your provider about your personal limits.

Questions to Ask Your Provider

How much walking or exercise is safe for me right now?

Is it safe for me to climb stairs or carry groceries?

When can I resume sexual activity?

Are there specific signs that mean I should stop what I'm doing (like dizziness or chest tightness)?

Can I play golf, garden, or travel once I feel stronger?

Should I wear compression stockings or avoid certain positions?

Patient Perspective: "I only plan one activity a day – like making dinner or meeting a friend. Anything more wipes me out. "I'm constantly tired. Even little things feel big now. You have to accept limits – it's hard, but it's reality."

Eating for a Healthier Heart

Limit Sodium (Salt)

- ☐ Aim for less than 2,000 mg per day (Keep in mind— 1 teaspoon of table salt = 2,300 mg of sodium).
- ☐ Avoid processed meats, canned soups, fast food, and salty snacks.
- ☐ Use herbs, lemon, or vinegar for flavor instead of salt.

Watch Fluids

- ☐ Some people need to limit total fluids to about 2 liters (about 8 cups) per day.
- ☐ Count everything that's liquid — water, coffee, soup, gelatin, and ice.
- ☐ Ask your provider what your personal limit should be.

Notes:

Heart-Healthy Foods

- ☐ Choose more fruits, vegetables, whole grains, lean proteins, and healthy fats (olive oil, nuts, fish).
- ☐ Limit alcohol; even small amounts can strain your heart or interact with medications.
- ☐ I know a Registered Dietitian who may be able to help you: https://www.simplehealthoptions.com/

Patient perspective: "I used to salt everything — even fruit! Now I keep herbs and lemon juice on the counter. It took me a few weeks, but my taste buds adjusted."

Sample 3-Day Heart-Healthy, Low-Sodium Meal Plan

Simple, affordable foods to support heart health and reduce fluid buildup.

Day 1

Breakfast:

- ½ cup dry oatmeal made with water, topped with ½ banana and cinnamon
- 1 boiled egg
- 1 cup black coffee or unsweetened tea

Snack:

- Small apple or pear

Lunch:

- Tuna salad made with 3 oz tuna (no-salt-added), 1 tbsp light mayo, chopped celery, and black pepper
- 2 slices low-sodium whole-grain bread
- 1 small side salad with olive oil + vinegar

Snack:

- Unsalted almonds (about ¼ cup)

Dinner:

- 3–4 oz baked or grilled chicken breast with garlic and herbs
- ½ cup brown rice
- 1 cup steamed green beans
- 1 small orange or clementine

Approximate sodium: 1,400–1,600 mg

Day 2

Breakfast:

- 1 slice whole-grain toast with 1 tbsp peanut butter (unsalted)
- ½ cup low-fat milk or calcium-fortified almond milk
- ½ cup berries

Snack:

- Carrot sticks or cucumber slices

Lunch:

- 1 cup homemade vegetable soup (low-sodium broth or no added salt)
- ½ turkey sandwich: 2 oz low-sodium turkey, lettuce, tomato, mustard
- 1 small apple

Snack:

- Greek yogurt (plain, low-fat) with cinnamon or fruit

Dinner:

- 3 oz baked salmon or tilapia with lemon and dill
- ½ cup mashed sweet potatoes
- 1 cup steamed broccoli
- 1 small piece of fruit (grapes or melon)

Approximate sodium: 1,500–1,800 mg

Day 3

Breakfast:

- 2 scrambled eggs (no salt added) with spinach and tomato
- 1 slice whole-grain toast
- ½ grapefruit

Snack:

- Unsalted popcorn (about 3 cups)

Lunch:

- ½ cup cooked beans (black or kidney, rinsed) over ½ cup brown rice
- 1 small salad with olive oil and vinegar
- 1 piece of fruit (pear or apple)

Snack:

- Low-fat string cheese or 1 oz unsalted nuts

Dinner:

- 3 oz lean pork tenderloin or skinless chicken thigh
- ½ cup quinoa or couscous
- 1 cup roasted vegetables (zucchini, peppers, onion)
- 1 baked apple with cinnamon

Approximate sodium: 1,600 mg

Small food swaps add up to less swelling and more energy–Stacie the PA

Some good tips from a dietitian:

☐ **Avoid adding salt** when cooking — flavor with lemon, herbs, onion, garlic, or vinegar.

☐ **Rinse canned beans and veggies** before using to remove extra sodium.

☐ **Limit sauces** like soy, teriyaki, or BBQ — even “light” versions can be high in sodium.

☐ **Fluid control:** If you have a daily fluid limit, remember that milk, soups, gelatin, and even ice count toward that total.

☐ **Grocery tip:** Store brands often have lower-sodium “no salt added” versions that are cheaper than national brands.

Finding Your Salt Balance

- Very strict sodium limits (below 2,000 mg) aren't necessary for everyone.
- Focus on avoiding processed and restaurant foods, reading labels, and finding a sustainable goal that keeps swelling down and food enjoyable.

(*Based on the SODIUM-HF study, 2022.*)

Eating Out Guide: Enjoying Restaurants with Heart Failure

- Having heart failure doesn't mean giving up your favorite restaurants — it just means learning how to make smarter choices.
- Restaurant food is one of the biggest hidden sources of salt and calories, but a few small changes can keep your meal heart-friendly and still enjoyable.

Before You Go

☐ **Check the menu online.** Most chains list nutrition info — look for items under 600 mg sodium per entrée.

☐ **Eat a small snack first.** A piece of fruit or a few unsalted nuts helps prevent overeating or ordering high-salt foods when you're starving.

☐ **Drink water early.** Sip slowly, and skip refills if you have a fluid limit.

At the Table

- ☐ **Tell your server:**
  "I'm on a low-salt diet — please ask the cook not to add salt, sauces, or butter." Most restaurants are used to this request.

- ☐ **Ask for sauces and dressings on the side.**
  Dip your fork in the dressing instead of pouring it.

- ☐ **Avoid the breadbasket and chips.**
  Bread, crackers, and chips are surprisingly high in sodium and can trigger fluid buildup.

- ☐ **Choose baked, grilled, or steamed foods.**
  Fried foods and sauces add salt, oil, and calories.

- ☐ **Add flavor, not salt:**
  Ask for lemon, pepper, or vinegar. Avoid soy sauce, teriyaki, BBQ, and broth-based gravies.

Smarter Choices by Cuisine

American / Diner Food:

- ☐ Choose grilled chicken, fish, or turkey burger without cheese or bacon.

- ☐ Skip fries; order fruit, baked potato (plain), or side salad with oil & vinegar.

Mexican:

- ☐ Choose grilled fajitas or tacos with corn tortillas, not enchiladas or burritos drowned in sauce.
- ☐ Ask for no added cheese or sour cream, and go easy on the chips.
- ☐ Use fresh salsa or pico de gallo for flavor — they're lower in sodium than sauces.

Italian:

- ☐ Choose red sauce over creamy Alfredo.
- ☐ Ask for light sauce and no added salt or cheese on top.
- ☐ Try grilled chicken, seafood, or whole-grain pasta with veggies.

Asian (Chinese, Thai, Japanese):

- ☐ Ask for steamed dishes with sauce on the side.
- ☐ Request "no MSG or added salt."
- ☐ Use just a small drizzle of soy or teriyaki sauce — each tablespoon has about 1,000 mg of sodium!

Sandwich or Sub Shop:

- ☐ Choose turkey or grilled chicken (not deli ham or salami).
- ☐ Load up on veggies; skip pickles, cheese, and condiments.
- ☐ Choose mustard over mayo, and ask for "no added salt or seasoning."

Fast Food:

- ☐ Order the smallest size possible.
- ☐ Choose grilled over fried.
- ☐ Skip cheese, bacon, and salty toppings.
- ☐ Ask for no salt on fries — or share one small portion.

When You Get Home

- **Weigh yourself the next morning.**
  If you're up more than 2–3 pounds, your meal may have been too salty. Drink plain water and return to your usual low-sodium meals the next day.

- **Don't feel guilty — just reset.**
  Everyone splurges sometimes; the key is getting back on track quickly.

Quick Restaurant Rules of Thumb

- ☐ "Fresh" beats "fried."
- ☐ "Grilled" beats "smothered."
- ☐ "Sauce on the side" beats "extra sauce."
- ☐ "Ask questions" beats "assume."

- Eating well isn't just about what's on your plate — it's also about how you feel.

- Making healthy choices day after day can be exhausting, especially when you're living with heart failure.

- That's why caring for your emotional health is just as important as caring for your heart.

- Learning to manage stress, sleep better, and practice mindfulness can help you stay on track with your goals and feel more in control of your health journey.

Emotional Health and Stress Management

Living with heart failure can be emotional. It's normal to feel anxious, frustrated, or afraid.

High stress levels can raise blood pressure and heart rate, so managing stress is part of treatment.

Try:

- Deep breathing or mindfulness exercises
- Talking with a counselor or joining a support group
- Gentle yoga or stretching (if cleared by your provider)
- Connecting with friends and family regularly

If sadness or worry lasts for weeks, tell your provider — treatment for anxiety or depression can greatly improve recovery.

Patient Perspective: "My husband is amazing. He's taken over the heavy cleaning and helps me with everything. Support makes all the difference. I don't know how I'd manage without him. My faith and my family keep me going. The church has been wonderful. My granddaughters still need me. I want to be in their lives as long as I can."

Sleep and Rest

- Fatigue is common with heart failure.
- Aim for 7–9 hours of sleep per night, and elevate your head slightly if shortness of breath worsens when lying flat.
- If you snore loudly or wake up gasping, ask about testing for **sleep apnea**, which is common in heart-failure patients and treatable.

Staying on Track

- **Weigh yourself every morning** after using the bathroom and before breakfast.
  Write it down — a sudden gain of 2–3 pounds in 24 hours or 5 pounds in a week may mean fluid is returning.

- **Take medications exactly as prescribed.** Don't skip doses.

- **Keep all follow-up appointments** — small medication changes make big differences.

- **Carry a medication list** and your cardiologist's contact info everywhere.

- **Get flu and pneumonia vaccines** to protect your lungs and heart.

Practical Tools and Home Tips for Living with Heart Failure

- Living with heart failure doesn't always mean buying expensive equipment.

- A few small changes at home can make daily life easier, safer, and more comfortable — especially when shortness of breath or fatigue make simple tasks harder.

Daily Monitoring Tools

- ☐ **Digital Scale:** Weigh yourself every morning after using the bathroom. Record it right away — a gain of 2–3 lbs in a day or 5 lbs in a week is a red flag.

- ☐ **Automatic Blood Pressure Cuff:** Choose an upper-arm model with a large, easy-read screen. Check once daily and record the reading in your weight log.

- ☐ **Pulse Oximeter (Optional):** Clips on your finger to measure oxygen level and pulse rate. Can help track shortness of breath episodes.

- ☐ **Medication Organizer:** Weekly pillboxes or automatic dispensers help prevent missed doses.

- ☐ **Notebook or App for Tracking:** Record weight, BP, HR, swelling, and any new symptoms — bring this to every appointment.

Helpful Home Comfort Aids

- ☐ **Reclining Chair or Adjustable Bed:**
  Helps keep your upper body elevated if lying flat makes you

short of breath.

- ☐ **Extra Pillows or a Wedge Pillow:** Reduces nighttime shortness of breath (orthopnea).

- ☐ **Shower Chair and Handheld Shower Head:** Conserve energy and reduce the risk of falls when bathing.

- ☐ **Raised Toilet Seat or Grab Bars:** Makes it easier to stand up without straining.

- ☐ **Non-Slip Mats and Good Lighting:** Prevents falls and allows safe movement during fatigue spells.

- ☐ **Lightweight Cleaning Tools or Reach Grabber:** Helps you do household chores without bending or lifting.

- ☐ **Compression Stockings (if recommended):** Can help with mild leg swelling — only under your provider's direction.

Notes:

____

____

____

____

Technology That Can Help

☐ **Remote Monitoring Apps or Bluetooth Scales:**
Some clinics link your scale or BP cuff to a phone app so readings go straight to your care team.

☐ **Smart Pill Caps or Reminders:**
Timers, beeps, or phone alerts can help you take medications on time.

☐ **Home Blood Pressure/Weight Sharing:**
Ask your provider if they can monitor your readings electronically between visits.

Energy-Saving Tips

☐ Keep essential items waist-high to avoid bending or reaching.

☐ Sit while dressing, cooking, or shaving.

☐ Break chores into smaller steps with rest breaks in between.

☐ Keep a chair in the kitchen or hallway for quick rests.

☐ Use rolling carts or baskets to carry groceries instead of lifting.

Notes:

Living Better with Heart Failure: Practical Everyday Tips

- Living with heart failure means finding ways to stay steady, strong, and supported.
- You can't control everything about the condition — but you can control your daily routine and your environment.
- These small steps add up to fewer flare-ups and more good days.

---

1. Keep a Daily Routine

☐ Take medicines at the **same time every day.** Use a pill organizer or phone alarm.

☐ **Weigh yourself and check your blood pressure** each morning. Record it in a notebook or app.

☐ Eat meals at regular times to avoid skipped doses or low energy.

☐ Go to bed and wake up on a steady schedule — your heart likes rhythm.

---

2. Move Every Day — But Pace Yourself

☐ Light walking, stretching, or chair yoga can strengthen your heart and muscles.

☐ Spread chores throughout the day. Rest before you feel exhausted.

☐ Try “energy zoning”: keep chairs or stools in spots where you often need a rest (like the kitchen or hallway).

☐ If cleared by your provider, join a **cardiac rehab maintenance class** — even once a week helps.

---

3. Keep Your Home “Heart Friendly”

☐ **Avoid extremes of heat or cold** — both strain the heart.

☐ **Stay cool in summer:** use a fan or light layers; avoid working outdoors during the hottest part of the day.

☐ **Stay warm in winter:** wear layers instead of cranking up heat; sudden temperature changes can trigger shortness of breath.

☐ **Reduce clutter and trip hazards.** A clear path means less energy wasted and fewer falls.

☐ **Keep things waist-high** so you’re not bending or reaching.

☐ Keep bottled or filtered water handy so you can sip small amounts throughout the day instead of large gulps.

---

4. Manage Fluids Wisely

- ☐ Follow your provider's daily limit (often about 2 liters).
- ☐ Use a **measured refillable bottle** so you know exactly how much you drink.
- ☐ Flavor water with lemon or mint instead of sugary drinks.
- ☐ Watch for "hidden fluids": soups, ice cream, gelatin, and even juicy fruits count.

---

5. Protect Yourself from Illness

- ☐ Get yearly **flu** and **COVID-19** shots, plus **pneumonia, RSV, and shingles** vaccines as advised.
- ☐ Wash hands frequently.
- ☐ Keep masks handy for crowded indoor areas or cold/flu season.
- ☐ Ask visitors who are sick to come another day.
- ☐ Treat fevers or infections early — they can trigger a heart-failure flare-up.

---

6. Emotional and Mental Health

- ☐ Talk openly about anxiety, fear, or frustration — you're not alone.
- ☐ Join a local or online **support group** (AHA, Mended Hearts, or hospital programs).
- ☐ Practice **relaxation breathing**: inhale slowly for 4 seconds, hold for 2, exhale for 6.
- ☐ Set small goals and celebrate progress — like walking a few extra minutes or cooking a healthy meal.

---

7. For Family and Caregivers

- ☐ Learn the patient's "baseline": their normal weight, breathing, and energy.
- ☐ Keep a shared notebook or phone note for symptoms, weights, and medications.
- ☐ Know the **red-flag signs** (rapid weight gain, shortness of breath, swelling, confusion) and when to call the provider.
- ☐ Encourage gentle activity but respect fatigue.
- ☐ Take turns caregiving — burnout helps no one.
- ☐ Ask for **respite care or home-health support** if the load gets heavy.

8. Plan for the Future — Early and Calmly

- ☐ Update **advance directives** when you're well, not in crisis.
- ☐ Discuss what treatments you'd want if symptoms worsen — it's about peace of mind, not giving up.
- ☐ Know that **palliative care** is about comfort and living better, not just end-of-life care.

---

9. Stay Curious and Engaged

- ☐ Ask questions at every appointment: "What can I do at home to help?"
- ☐ Bring your logs and symptom notes to show patterns.
- ☐ Keep learning — the more you understand your heart, the more power you have to protect it.

Notes:

Key Takeaway

- Cardiac rehab and mindful daily habits can dramatically improve strength, mood, and quality of life.
- Small steps — steady exercise, healthy food choices, stress control, and honest talks with your care team — build the best foundation for long-term heart health.
- The secret to living longer and better with heart failure isn't one big change — it's dozens of small, steady habits.
- A safe home, a clear routine, good sleep, and honest communication with your care team can make all the difference.
- You can still enjoy dining out while protecting your heart — it's all about *asking, choosing, and portioning.*
- With a few small requests and smart swaps, you'll walk away satisfied and in control of your heart health.
- The best "assistive devices" for heart failure are those that keep you safe, prevent fatigue, and help you notice changes early.
- Small investments — a reliable scale, BP cuff, and safe home setup — can save hospital visits and improve comfort every single day.
- Eating for heart failure doesn't mean bland or expensive meals.
- Simple home-cooked foods with fresh or frozen produce, lean proteins, and spices can taste great, reduce swelling, and support your heart every day.

References

American College of Cardiology (ACC), American Heart Association (AHA), Heart Failure Society of America (HFSA) Guidelines 2022–2024; *Circulation*, 2023; *UpToDate*, reviewed 2025; *National Heart, Lung, and Blood Institute (NHLBI)*, 2024.

Key Terms for this Section:

Activity Tolerance:
How much movement or exercise you can do before feeling short of breath, tired, or dizzy.

Blood Pressure:
The force of blood against the artery walls. High blood pressure makes the heart work harder.

Cardiac Rehabilitation (Cardiac Rehab):
A supervised program that includes exercise, education, and counseling to help people recover from heart problems and improve heart strength.

Compression Stockings:
Special socks that gently squeeze the legs to prevent swelling and improve circulation.

Depression:
A medical condition that causes ongoing sadness, low energy, and loss of interest in normal activities. Common after heart problems and treatable.

Dietitian:
A healthcare professional who helps patients plan healthy, low-sodium, heart-friendly meals.

Fluid Restriction:
A limit on how much fluid (including drinks and soups) a person can have each day to prevent swelling and fluid overload.

Fluids:
Any liquid you drink or eat in soft form, such as water, coffee, tea, milk, soup, gelatin, or ice.

Heart-Healthy Diet:
A way of eating that includes fruits, vegetables, whole grains, lean proteins, and healthy fats while limiting salt, sugar, and

saturated fats.

Mindfulness:
A relaxation technique that focuses on slow breathing and being aware of the present moment to reduce stress.

Pacing:
Balancing activity and rest so you don't overexert yourself.

Sexual Activity:
Physical intimacy that raises the heart rate; usually safe when you can climb two flights of stairs or walk briskly without shortness of breath or chest pain.

Sleep Apnea:
A sleep disorder that causes brief pauses in breathing at night, leading to poor rest and strain on the heart.

Sodium (Salt):
A mineral found in many foods that causes the body to retain fluid; should be limited to about 2,000 mg per day in most heart-failure patients.

Stress Management:
Ways to reduce mental tension, such as deep breathing, light exercise, hobbies, or talking with a counselor.

Support Group:
A group of people who share similar experiences and provide encouragement and advice to each other.

Vaccinations:
Shots that help protect against illnesses like the flu or pneumonia, which can be more serious in heart-failure patients.

Weight Tracking:
Daily weighing to detect early fluid buildup; a sudden increase of 2–3 pounds in a day or 5 pounds in a week may mean worsening heart failure.

SECTION 8

Hospital and ICU Care

What to Expect During a Heart Failure Stay

Most people with heart failure never need intensive care. But if it happens, here's what to expect so it feels less frightening– Stacie the PA

Being admitted to the hospital for heart failure can feel overwhelming.

Knowing what to expect — the people, machines, medicines, and next-step decisions — can make the experience less frightening and help you take an active role in your recovery.

Why Patients Are Hospitalized for Heart Failure

Most hospital stays happen when symptoms suddenly worsen, such as:

- Severe shortness of breath or fluid in the lungs
- Swelling that doesn't improve with home medicines
- Very high or very low blood pressure
- Irregular or fast heartbeat (arrhythmia)
- New or worsening kidney problems

The goal is to remove excess fluid, stabilize your breathing and heart rhythm, and find out *why* the flare-up happened.

Common Treatments in the Hospital

Treatment	Purpose	How Long It's Used
IV Diuretics (furosemide/Lasix®, bumetanide/Bumex®)	Pull extra fluid out of the body quickly	Until swelling and breathing improve (usually 1–3 days)
IV Vasodilators (nitroglycerin, nesiritide)	Relax blood vessels and lower pressure on the heart	Short-term; stopped once stable
IV Inotropes (dobutamine, milrinone)	Help a very weak heart pump stronger	Used only in severe cases or ICU
Oxygen or CPAP/BiPAP	Ease shortness of breath	Until oxygen levels return to normal
Heparin or other blood thinners	Prevent clots during bed rest	While hospitalized
Electrolyte replacements (potassium, magnesium)	Keep heart rhythm stable	As needed

Understanding ICU Monitors and Machines

If you or your loved one need intensive care, you'll see several machines that track how your heart and lungs are working.

Monitor or Device	What It Measures	What It Tells the Team
EKG Monitor	Heart rate and rhythm	Detects arrhythmias or heart strain
Blood Pressure (MAP)	Mean Arterial Pressure — the average blood pressure over time	Ensures organs are getting enough blood flow
Oxygen Monitor (Pulse Ox)	Oxygen level in the blood	Confirms oxygen therapy is working
CVP (Central Venous Pressure)	Pressure inside large chest veins	Shows how much fluid is in your system
BNP or NT-proBNP Lab	Hormone level from the heart	Helps track improvement or worsening heart strain
IV Pump	Delivers fluids and medications safely	Controls medicine speed and dose

You may also see **nasal oxygen tubing**, **urinary catheter**, or **small IV lines** for medications — all temporary and removed once stable.

Patient Perspective: "All those beeps and wires looked terrifying at first, but the nurses explained every one. Once I understood what each monitor did, it didn't feel so scary."

Deciding on Procedures Before You Leave the Hospital

While you recover, your care team will evaluate whether additional procedures could help prevent future hospital stays.

- **Valve Repair or Replacement:** Recommended if a leaking or narrowed valve is making your heart work too hard.

Many valve procedures can be done through a catheter (TAVR or MitraClip) instead of open surgery.

- **Pacemaker or Cardiac Resynchronization Therapy (CRT):** Helps the heart's chambers beat together more effectively.

- **Implantable Defibrillator (ICD):** Prevents sudden cardiac arrest if your heart has a dangerous rhythm.

- **Right-Heart Catheterization:** Sometimes done before discharge to measure internal pressures and guide medication adjustments.

Your provider will discuss the risks, benefits, and timing for any of these options.

Remote Monitoring Option

- If you are hospitalized often for fluid buildup, your provider may suggest a small implanted pressure sensor (CardioMEMS®).
- It monitors your heart pressure from home so your team can adjust medications early and prevent readmission.

The ICU Team: Who's in the Room

Team Member	Role in Your Care
Cardiologist or Heart Failure Specialist	Leads medical decisions and treatment plan
Intensivist or Hospitalist	Oversees daily care in the ICU or hospital ward
Advanced Practice Provider (PA / NP)	Examines you daily, manages medications, coordinates discharge
Nurses	Monitor vital signs, give medicines, and provide education
Respiratory Therapist	Manages oxygen, CPAP, or ventilator settings
Pharmacist	Reviews medications for safety and interactions
Dietitian	Helps plan low-sodium, heart-healthy meals
Social Worker or Case Manager	Arranges follow-up appointments, home health, and equipment

Common ICU Terms You Might Hear

Term	Meaning
MAP (Mean Arterial Pressure)	A steady measure of blood flow to the organs; usually kept above 65 mm Hg.
CVP (Central Venous Pressure)	Reflects how much fluid is in the veins returning to the heart.
BNP / NT-proBNP	Lab markers that rise when the heart is stressed.
Telemetry	Continuous heart-rhythm monitoring on a portable unit.
Inotrope	A medicine that helps the heart contract more strongly.
Diuresis	The process of removing fluid through urination, often with IV "water pills."

Going Home After a Hospital Stay

Before discharge, your team will:

- Adjust medications for home use.
- Review your **daily weight**, **salt**, and **fluid** goals.
- Schedule **follow-up visits** within 7 days.
- Recommend **cardiac rehab** or light activity once stable.
- Explain new devices or procedures, if done.

Key Takeaway

- Hospital stays for heart failure are usually short and focused on getting fluid off, balancing medications, and identifying the cause of the flare-up.
- Knowing what to expect — and what all those tubes and monitors mean — can make your experience less stressful and your recovery faster.

References

American College of Cardiology (ACC), American Heart Association (AHA), Heart Failure Society of America (HFSA) Guidelines 2022–2024; *Circulation*, 2023; *Journal of the American College of Cardiology*, 2022–2024; *UpToDate*, reviewed 2025.

Key Terms for this Section

BNP (B-type Natriuretic Peptide):
A hormone released when the heart muscle is stretched or stressed. High levels often mean fluid buildup or worsening heart failure.

Cardiac Catheterization:
A procedure using thin tubes placed through a blood vessel to measure heart pressures or check for blockages.

Cardiac Resynchronization Therapy (CRT):
A special pacemaker that helps both sides of the heart beat together so it pumps more efficiently.

Case Manager / Social Worker:
A hospital professional who helps arrange follow-up visits, home health, and equipment before discharge.

Central Venous Pressure (CVP):
A measurement of fluid pressure in large chest veins that shows how much fluid is in the body.

Diuresis:
The medical term for removing extra fluid from the body, usually by using "water pills."

Ejection Fraction (EF):
The percentage of blood the left ventricle pumps out with each beat; a key measure of heart strength.

Electrolytes:
Minerals such as sodium, potassium, and magnesium that help control heart rhythm and muscle function.

ICD (Implantable Cardioverter-Defibrillator):
A small device placed in the chest that can shock or pace the heart if a dangerous rhythm occurs.

Inotrope:
A medicine that helps the heart contract more strongly when it is very weak.

Intensivist / Hospitalist:
A doctor who manages daily care for patients in the ICU or hospital unit.

IV (Venous Line):
A small tube placed in a vein to give fluids or medications directly into the bloodstream.

MAP (Mean Arterial Pressure):
The average blood pressure inside the arteries over time; shows whether organs are getting enough blood flow.

Nesiritide:
A short-term IV medicine that relaxes blood vessels and helps reduce heart-failure symptoms in the hospital.

Oxygen Saturation (Pulse Oximetry):
A measure of how much oxygen is in your blood; shown as a percentage on a fingertip monitor.

Telemetry:
Continuous heart-rhythm monitoring used in the hospital to watch for arrhythmias.

Vasodilator:
A medicine that relaxes and widens blood vessels to lower blood pressure and reduce strain on the heart.

❤ You're not alone.

Every recovery is different. These experiences are intense, but they're also temporary. With medical care, rest, and support, most people regain their independence — and often, a new appreciation for life.

SECTION 9

Long-Term Planning

and

Home Health

Having a Plan Matters

Heart failure is a long-term condition, and your care plan may change over time. This section helps you to be more prepared, so you stay independent, make your wishes known, and keep your quality of life as high as possible.

Home Health and Ongoing Care

After a hospital stay or as symptoms change, your provider may recommend **home health services**. These are designed to help you stay safe and supported at home.

Home health may include:

- Regular nurse visits to check blood pressure, weight, and medications
- Physical therapy to help you move safely and build strength
- Education on diet, fluid limits, and recognizing early warning signs
- Coordination between your home team and your cardiologist

You can still see your regular provider while receiving home health — it's an *extension* of your care, not a replacement.

Patient Perspective: "Having the nurse come by once a week gave me peace of mind. It's not just medical — they notice things I miss, like swelling or weight changes."

When to Consider Palliative Care

Palliative care focuses on comfort, quality of life, and symptom relief — *not just end-of-life care.*

It can be started **at any stage** of heart failure, especially if you have:

- Frequent hospitalizations
- Worsening shortness of breath or fatigue
- Multiple medications with complex schedules
- Emotional or spiritual distress related to illness

Palliative care can help with:

- Adjusting medications to reduce symptoms
- Managing anxiety or depression
- Talking through goals and treatment preferences with your family
- Coordinating between your cardiologist, primary care, and home services

Many heart-failure patients use palliative care for years as part of living well — not just in the final stages.

Hospice Care (When Heart Failure Becomes Advanced)

If the heart becomes too weak to respond to treatment and symptoms are difficult to control, **hospice** may be recommended.

Hospice provides expert comfort care at home or in a dedicated center, focusing on dignity, symptom control, and family support.

The hospice team includes:

- Nurses available 24/7 for urgent needs
- Providers who manage medications for pain or shortness of breath
- Social workers and chaplains for emotional and spiritual support

You can stop or start hospice at any time — it's your choice.

The goal is to keep you comfortable, not to stop all care.

Notes:

Advance Directives and Medical Wishes

Having your wishes written down takes pressure off your loved ones and helps your care team follow your values. Having a DNR or living will is not 'giving up'—it tells your team how to honor your wishes.

Common forms include:

- **Living Will:** States what medical treatments you do or don't want (like CPR, intubation, or feeding tubes).
- **DNR (Do Not Resuscitate):** This tells emergency teams not to use CPR (or defibrillator-the shocker things) if your heart stops.
- **DNI (Do Not Intubate):** States that you don't want a breathing tube placed.
- **Healthcare Proxy (Medical Power of Attorney):** Names someone you trust to make medical decisions if you can't.

You can change these forms at any time.

Give copies to your provider, your family, and anyone likely to be present in an emergency.

Notes:

Discussing Goals of Care

Talking about your future care doesn't mean giving up — it means making your voice heard. Ask your provider to help you think about:

- What quality of life means to you
- What symptoms you find unacceptable or frightening
- What level of care you'd want in an emergency
- When you'd want comfort-focused care to take priority

Many patients find these discussions bring peace of mind, not fear.

The best time to make decisions is when you're *feeling well* and can clearly express your wishes.

Patient perspective: "I don't want to be on machines in a nursing home – that's not living to me. It's not black and white – it's about what kind of life you want to live. I had these conversations with my husband and I worry that he won't be able to let me go if it comes to it."

Notes:

Support for Families and Caregivers

Heart failure affects the whole household, not just the patient.

Family members often manage medications, meals, and appointments — and they need care, too.

Encourage your caregivers to:

- Take breaks and care for their own health
- Ask the medical team for clear instructions
- Join caregiver support groups (in-person or online)
- Seek respite care if they need time to rest

Remember, caring for yourself helps you care for your loved one.

Notes:

Questions to Ask Your Provider

Would home health or palliative care help me manage my symptoms better?

How will I know if it's time to consider hospice?

Who can help me complete a living will or healthcare proxy form?

What are the signs that my heart failure may be getting worse?

Can you help my family understand what to expect and how to help?

Key Takeaway

- Planning ahead isn't about giving up — it's about taking control, and allowing your family to **KNOW** what you would want instead of guessing (and feeling guilty about it).
- Understanding your options for home health, palliative care, and advance planning lets you and your family focus on what matters most: comfort, dignity, and time together.

Talking with Family and Documenting Wishes

- Conversations about end-of-life care are hard — but silence often leaves family members guessing.
- The best time to talk is now, before a crisis.

Notes:

Steps you can take:

1. Think about what matters most to you. Is it living as long as possible, staying at home, avoiding pain, or something else?

2. Choose a health care decision maker. Pick someone you trust to speak for you if you can't.

3. Share your wishes clearly. Use simple language: "If my heart stops, I want to be kept comfortable, not put on machines."

4. Put it in writing. Ask your provider for advance directive forms or living will templates.

5. Update it when needed. Review your choices after major health changes or hospital stays.

Notes:

My Care Preferences: Fill this out so you can start the conversation with your loved ones.

Topic	**My Wishes / Notes**
If my heart gets weaker, my biggest goal is…	
I would prefer to receive care at… (home, hospital, hospice, other)	
I would like these treatments if possible:	
I would **not** want these treatments:	
The person I trust to make medical decisions for me is…	
My provider's name and phone number:	
Where my advance directive or POLST/MOST forms are kept:	
My spiritual or emotional preferences:	
Other wishes (music, visitors, messages):	

References

American College of Cardiology (ACC), American Heart Association (AHA), Heart Failure Society of America (HFSA) Guidelines 2022–2024; *UpToDate*, reviewed 2025; *National Institute on Aging (NIA)*, 2024; *Centers for Medicare & Medicaid Services (CMS)*, 2025.

Key Terms for this Section

Advance Directive:
A legal document that states your medical care preferences if you become too sick to speak for yourself.

Caregiver:
A family member, friend, or hired helper who assists with daily care, medications, appointments, or emotional support.

Comfort Care:
Medical treatment focused on relieving symptoms and maintaining comfort, rather than curing disease.

CPR (Cardiopulmonary Resuscitation):
An emergency procedure that uses chest compressions and sometimes a defibrillator to restart the heart after cardiac arrest.

DNI (Do Not Intubate):
A medical order stating you do not want a breathing tube placed if your lungs fail.

DNR (Do Not Resuscitate):
A medical order that tells healthcare providers not to perform CPR if your heart stops.

Healthcare Proxy (Medical Power of Attorney):
A person you choose to make healthcare decisions for you if you cannot make them yourself.

Home Health:
A service that brings nurses, therapists, or other healthcare professionals to your home for ongoing monitoring and education.

Hospice Care:
A specialized program that provides comfort, pain control, and emotional support for people with advanced illness who are no longer pursuing aggressive treatments.

Living Will:
A written statement that explains what medical treatments you would or would not want if you were seriously ill or near the end of life.

Palliative Care:
A type of care focused on improving quality of life and controlling symptoms such as pain, fatigue, or shortness of breath at any stage of illness.

Respite Care:
Temporary relief for family caregivers — another professional or service steps in to provide care so the main caregiver can rest.

Social Worker:
A professional who helps coordinate resources, home services, financial aid, or counseling for patients and families.

Symptom Management:
Controlling distressing symptoms (such as shortness of breath, fatigue, or anxiety) to improve comfort and daily function.

Final Thought

"Preparing for tomorrow doesn't take away from today — it makes every heartbeat more meaningful." — Stacie the PA

SECTION 10

Living Well with Heart Failure

and

Helpful Resources

It CAN be Managed

- Heart failure is a serious condition, but it doesn't have to define your life.
- With the right care plan, daily habits, and support, many people live full, meaningful lives for years — working, traveling, and spending time with family and friends.
- The key is to understand your body, stay consistent with treatment, and know when to reach out for help.

Daily Habits That Make a Difference

Small, steady actions can prevent flare-ups and hospital visits.

- **Take medications exactly as prescribed.** Never skip doses or stop medicines suddenly.
- **Weigh yourself every morning.** A gain of 2–3 pounds in a day or 5 pounds in a week may mean fluid buildup.
- **Follow your sodium and fluid goals.** Too much salt or liquid makes the heart work harder.
- **Stay active safely.** Gentle exercise strengthens the heart, muscles, and mood.
- **Keep all follow-up visits.** Even if you feel well, routine check-ins prevent setbacks.
- **Get enough rest.** Fatigue means your body needs time to recover.
- **Report new symptoms early.** Don't wait — call your provider if you notice swelling, cough, or new shortness of breath.
- Monitor your **blood pressure and heart rate** daily.
  Call if your blood pressure is below 90/60 with dizziness or if your heart rate drops below 50 beats per minute.

Emotional and Mental Health

It's normal to feel frustrated or anxious after a diagnosis of heart failure. Managing your emotional health is part of your treatment.

Try:

- Talking with a counselor or support group — you are not alone.
- Mindfulness and breathing exercises to lower stress.
- Setting small, realistic goals each week.
- Celebrating progress — even small improvements in energy or activity count.

Your mental health and heart health work hand-in-hand. Treat both with care.

Patient perspective: "I used to think asking for help meant I was weak. Now I see it as teamwork — my providers, my husband, and I all play a part in keeping me well."

Staying Connected with Your Care Team

Think of your heart-failure team as partners in your long-term care. It may include:

- Your Cardiologist or heart failure specialist
- An Advanced Practice Provider-APP (PA or NP)
- Your Primary Care Provider
- Nurses and Pharmacists, Dietitians, Social Workers, and Physical Therapists

Keep a written or digital list of everyone's contact information and your medication list.

Bring this list to every appointment or hospital visit.

Knowing When to Call for Help

Call your provider as directed and likely: if you notice:

- Weight gain of more than 2–3 pounds in 24 hours or 5 pounds in a week
- Shortness of breath, especially when lying flat
- New or worsening swelling in your legs or abdomen
- Dizziness, fainting, or unusual fatigue
- Fast, pounding, or irregular heartbeat

Call **911 or emergency services immediately** if you have:

- Chest pain that lasts more than a few minutes
- Fainting or severe shortness of breath
- Sudden confusion or inability to stay awake

Early attention can prevent a crisis.

Living Fully and Looking Ahead

- Having heart failure means you must be mindful — but it doesn't mean giving up joy.
- You can still plan trips, enjoy hobbies, and celebrate milestones.
- Living well comes down to balance — activity, rest, and awareness.
- Many patients find meaning in helping others — joining a heart-failure support group, sharing their story, or mentoring new patients.

Your experience can inspire someone else to take control of their health.

Stay Up to Date on Vaccines

- Flu (yearly), COVID-19 (seasonal)
- Pneumococcal (PCV20 or PCV15 → PPSV23)
- RSV (ages 60+ or high-risk)
- Shingles (Shingrix®, ages 50+)
- Ask your Provider if any others apply to you.

These reduce infection risk that can trigger a heart-failure flare-up.

Helpful National Resources

Here are trusted organizations that offer education, tools, and support for people living with heart failure:

- **American Heart Association (AHA):**
  Heart Failure resources, symptom trackers, and patient stories.
  www.heart.org

- **Heart Failure Society of America (HFSA):**
  Patient handouts, lifestyle tips, and educational videos.
  www.hfsa.org/patient-hub

- **National Heart, Lung, and Blood Institute (NHLBI):**
  Research updates and easy-to-read heart health information.
  www.nhlbi.nih.gov

- **Centers for Disease Control and Prevention (CDC):**
  Information about heart failure prevention and living well.
  www.cdc.gov/heart-disease

- **Mended Hearts:**
  A national peer-support group for heart patients and families.
  www.mendedhearts.org

- **Medicare Home Health & Hospice Resources:**
  Information about coverage for home health, palliative, and hospice care.
  www.medicare.gov

Heart Failure Support Classes:
Ask your local hospital or cardiac rehab center about small group programs or online classes designed for patients with chronic heart failure. These sessions reinforce lifestyle tips, medication safety, and emotional support.

■ *Heart Failure Self-Check*

Want to learn more about your heart-failure status?

Visit:

- **Heart Failure Society of America Patient Hub:** www.hfsa.org/patient-hub
- **American Heart Association Heart Failure Quiz:** www.heart.org/heart-failure-quiz

Keep updated lists of your:

- Your **blood pressure** (goal often under 130/80)
- Your **BNP or NT-proBNP** (ask your provider)
- Your **Ejection Fraction (EF)** from your last echo
- Your **daily weight trend**
- Bring these numbers to each appointment. Your provider can review them and calculate your formal risk score (MAGGIC or Seattle model).

Patient Perspective: "Heart failure changed my pace, not my purpose. I still laugh, cook, travel, and live — just differently, and more intentionally."

Key Takeaway

- Heart failure is part of your life — not the end of it.
- By staying informed, following your treatment plan, and reaching out for help when needed, you can live a long, meaningful life with more good days ahead.
- The most powerful medicine is hope, consistency, and teamwork.
- With good care and follow-up, many people with heart failure keep living full, active lives.

References

American College of Cardiology (ACC), American Heart Association (AHA), Heart Failure Society of America (HFSA) Guidelines 2022–2024; *UpToDate*, reviewed 2025; *National Heart, Lung, and Blood Institute (NHLBI)*, 2024; *Centers for Disease Control and Prevention (CDC)*, 2024; *Heart Failure Society of America (HFSA) Patient Hub.*

Key Terms for this Section

American Heart Association (AHA):
A national organization that provides education, research, and support for patients with heart and blood vessel diseases.

Cardiac Team:
The group of healthcare professionals who help manage heart failure — usually includes a cardiologist, PA or NP, nurses, pharmacists, dietitians, and therapists.

Centers for Disease Control and Prevention (CDC):
A federal public-health agency that shares information about preventing and managing chronic diseases like heart failure.

Consistency:
Following your daily routine — taking medications, eating well, tracking weight — to keep heart failure under control.

Dietitian:
A healthcare professional who helps you plan heart-healthy, low-sodium meals.

Fluid Tracking:
Recording how much you drink each day to stay within your provider's recommended fluid limit.

Heart Failure Society of America (HFSA):
A professional organization that provides reliable patient education and support materials on living with heart failure.

Lifestyle Changes:
Healthy habits — like eating less salt, exercising safely, and reducing stress — that help the heart work more efficiently.

Mended Hearts:
A national support organization for people living with heart disease and their families.

Mindfulness:

A relaxation technique that uses breathing and awareness to reduce stress and improve focus and calmness.

National Heart, Lung, and Blood Institute (NHLBI):
A division of the National Institutes of Health that conducts and shares heart-health research and educational materials.

Palliative Care:
Medical care focused on comfort and quality of life for people living with serious illness.

Symptom Tracker:
A daily log to record your weight, swelling, energy level, and breathing so you and your provider can notice early warning signs.

Support Group:
A group of people with shared experiences who meet to offer encouragement and practical advice.

Team-Based Care:
A collaborative approach where doctors, PAs, NPs, nurses, and specialists all communicate to manage your heart health together.

Telehealth:
A medical visit done by phone or video — helpful for follow-up care or medication checks from home.

Weight Monitoring:
Weigh yourself every morning to watch for quick changes that may mean fluid buildup.

Heart Failure Emergency Quick Reference

When you live with heart failure, small changes can become serious quickly.
Knowing when to call for help — and when to call 911 — can save your life.
Keep this page somewhere visible at home. Or tear it out and put on the fridge.

Call 911 or Go to the Nearest Emergency Room If You Have (or are not sure you have):

- Severe **shortness of breath** that does not improve with rest or oxygen
- **Chest pain or pressure** lasting more than a few minutes
- **Fainting**, confusion, or inability to stay awake
- **Coughing up pink, frothy sputum** (a sign of fluid in the lungs)
- **Sudden swelling** of the face, neck, or belly
- **Heart rate over 120 beats per minute** or irregular pounding that makes you lightheaded
- **Blue or gray skin color** around lips or fingertips
- **Severe weakness or inability to walk across a room** without gasping for air

Do not drive yourself.
Call 911 and bring your medication list, recent weights, and any recent test results with you.

📞 Call Your Provider Within 24 Hours If You Notice:

- Weight gain of **2–3 pounds in 24 hours** or **5 pounds in one week**
- New or worsening **swelling** in feet, ankles, legs, or belly
- Increased **fatigue, shortness of breath, or cough**
- **Trouble sleeping** or needing extra pillows to breathe comfortably
- **Dizziness, nausea, or decreased appetite**
- Feeling that your medications are **not working as well as before**

These may be early signs of fluid buildup or medication changes that need attention.

🩺 Keep These Numbers Handy:

Cardiologist: ______________________________

Primary Care Provider: ______________________
After-Hours / On-Call Number: _________________

Nearest Emergency Room: ______________________________

Preferred Hospital: ______________________________________

Before You Go to the Hospital

If possible, bring:

- A **current medication list** (name, dose, schedule)
- Your **latest weight log**
- Any **recent test results** or discharge papers
- Contact info for your **healthcare proxy or family member**

Stay Prepared

- Keep a **small packed bag** in case you need to go to the hospital.
- Update your **medication list** after every appointment.
- Post emergency numbers near your phone or refrigerator.
- Share this plan with family or caregivers.

Key Reminder: Most heart failure emergencies can be prevented by noticing early changes and acting quickly.
If something feels "off," trust your instincts — it's always safer to call.

Quick Daily Checklist

Every Morning

- ☐ Weigh myself after using the bathroom
- ☐ Take my medicines
- ☐ Check swelling and shortness of breath

Every Week

- ☐ Review sodium goals
- ☐ Refill prescriptions

Every Month

- ☐ Review weights and symptoms with provider

Patients love tear-out or fridge-magnet–style pages like this.

Glossary of Terms

A

ACE Inhibitor (Angiotensin-Converting Enzyme Inhibitor):
A medicine that helps relax blood vessels, lower blood pressure, and make it easier for the heart to pump.

Acute Heart Failure:
A sudden worsening of heart failure symptoms, such as shortness of breath or swelling, often requiring hospitalization.

Advance Directive:
A legal form that states your medical wishes if you become too sick to speak for yourself.

Aldosterone Antagonist:
A medication that removes extra salt and water from the body while helping the heart work more efficiently.

Aortic Valve:
The heart valve that controls blood flow from the left ventricle to the aorta (the main artery to the body).

Arrhythmia:
An abnormal heart rhythm — too fast, too slow, or irregular.

ARNI (Angiotensin Receptor–Neprilysin Inhibitor):
A modern heart-failure medication that combines two drugs to improve heart function and reduce strain.

B

Beta-Blocker:
A medicine that slows the heart rate and lowers blood pressure to reduce the heart's workload.

BNP (B-type Natriuretic Peptide):
A hormone released by the heart when it's stretched or stressed; high levels suggest heart failure or fluid buildup.

Blood Pressure:
The force of blood pushing against artery walls. High blood pressure can damage the heart over time.

Body Mass Index (BMI):
A measure of body fat based on height and weight; used to assess healthy weight range.

C

Calcium Scoring CT:
A scan that measures calcium buildup in artery walls to estimate future heart-disease risk.

Cardiac Catheterization:
A test using thin tubes to check for blockages or measure pressure inside the heart.

Cardiac Output:
The amount of blood pumped by the heart each minute.

Cardiac Rehabilitation (Cardiac Rehab):
A supervised program that includes exercise, education, and counseling to help people recover from heart problems.

Cardiologist:
A doctor who specializes in diagnosing and treating heart conditions.

Cardiomyopathy:
A disease of the heart muscle that weakens or stiffens the heart, making it harder to pump blood.

Cholesterol:
A waxy substance found in the blood; too much "bad" cholesterol (LDL) can block arteries.

CPR (Cardiopulmonary Resuscitation):
An emergency procedure that uses chest compressions to restart the heart when it stops beating.

CRT (Cardiac Resynchronization Therapy):
A special pacemaker that helps both sides of the heart beat in sync to pump more effectively.

CVP (Central Venous Pressure):
A measurement of the fluid pressure in large chest veins that helps monitor hydration and heart strain.

D

Depression:
A medical condition that causes sadness, fatigue, and loss of interest in normal activities; treatable with therapy or medication.

Diastolic Dysfunction:
A problem where the heart muscle is too stiff to fill properly between beats (seen in HFpEF).

Diuretic ("Water Pill"):
A medication that helps remove extra salt and water from the body to reduce swelling and shortness of breath.

DNI (Do Not Intubate):
A medical order stating you do not want a breathing tube placed if your lungs fail.

DNR (Do Not Resuscitate):
A medical order that tells providers not to perform CPR if your heart stops.

E

Echocardiogram (Echo):
An ultrasound test that shows how the heart's chambers, valves, and pumping function work in real time.

Ejection Fraction (EF):
The percentage of blood the left ventricle pumps out with each beat; normal is 50–70%.

Electrocardiogram (EKG or ECG):
A test that records the heart's electrical activity to detect rhythm problems or past heart attacks.

Entresto®:
A brand-name ARNI medication (sacubitril/valsartan) used to improve heart function in heart failure.

F

Family History:
Heart disease or heart failure in close relatives, which increases your own risk.

Fluid Restriction:
A limit on how much fluid a person can drink each day to prevent swelling and shortness of breath.

G

Gestational Diabetes:
High blood sugar that develops during pregnancy and raises long-term heart risk.

H

Heart Failure (HF):
A condition where the heart can't pump enough blood to meet the body's needs.

Heart Failure with Preserved Ejection Fraction (HFpEF):
A form of heart failure where the heart pumps normally but is too stiff to fill well.

Heart Failure with Reduced Ejection Fraction (HFrEF):
A form of heart failure where the heart muscle is weak and doesn't pump out enough blood.

Heart Valve:
A flap that opens and closes to control blood flow through the heart's chambers.

Healthcare Proxy (Medical Power of Attorney):
A person you choose to make healthcare decisions for you if you can't make them yourself.

Home Health:
Nursing and therapy services provided in your home to support recovery and manage chronic illness.

Hospice Care:
Comfort care for people with serious illness when treatment is no longer helping and focus shifts to quality of life.

Hypertension:
High blood pressure makes the heart work harder and increases heart failure risk.

Hypertrophic Cardiomyopathy:
A thickened heart muscle that limits blood flow and may cause chest pain or fainting.

I

ICD (Implantable Cardioverter-Defibrillator):
A small device that corrects dangerous heart rhythms by sending an electric shock.

Inotrope:
A medicine that helps the heart contract more strongly when it's very weak.

Ischemic Cardiomyopathy:
Heart muscle weakness caused by poor blood flow or prior heart attacks.

L

Left Ventricular Assist Device (LVAD):
A mechanical pump that helps a failing heart move blood to the body.

Lifestyle Changes:
Healthy habits such as eating less salt, exercising safely, and reducing stress to protect heart function.

Living Will:
A written statement describing the medical treatments you would or would not want if you become seriously ill.

M

MAP (Mean Arterial Pressure):
The average pressure in the arteries during one heartbeat cycle. It helps ensure organs are getting enough blood.

Medication Adherence:
Taking medicines exactly as prescribed, at the right dose and time.

Menopause:
The natural end of menstrual cycles, after which estrogen levels drop and heart risk increases.

Mindfulness:
A relaxation practice that focuses on breathing and awareness to reduce stress.

Mitral Valve:
The valve between the left atrium and ventricle; controls blood flow into the ventricle.

O

Oxygen Therapy:
Supplemental oxygen used to help with shortness of breath or low oxygen levels.

P

Pacemaker:
A small implanted device that regulates or stimulates the heartbeat.

Palliative Care:
Medical care focused on improving comfort and quality of life at any stage of illness.

Peripartum Cardiomyopathy:
Heart weakness that occurs during late pregnancy or soon after delivery.

Pulmonic Valve:
The valve between the right ventricle and pulmonary artery that controls blood flow to the lungs.

R

Restrictive Cardiomyopathy:
A rare type of heart disease where the heart muscle becomes stiff and can't fill easily.

Respite Care:
Short-term relief for caregivers when another person or service provides care temporarily.

S

SGLT2 Inhibitors:
Medicines that help the kidneys remove sugar and water; proven to improve outcomes in heart-failure patients.

Sleep Apnea:
A condition where breathing stops and starts during sleep, often worsening heart strain.

Sodium (Salt):
A mineral that causes the body to hold onto water; reducing sodium helps control swelling and blood pressure.

Stenosis:
A narrowing of a heart valve that makes it harder for blood to flow forward.

Stress Management:
Techniques such as deep breathing or light exercise that help reduce mental tension.

Support Group:
A group of people who share similar experiences and offer advice and encouragement.

Symptom Tracker:
A tool to record daily weight, swelling, or energy changes to spot early signs of worsening heart failure.

T

Telemetry:
A hospital system that continuously monitors heart rate and rhythm.

Testosterone:
A male hormone that affects muscle and heart health; levels naturally decrease with age.

Tricuspid Valve:
The valve between the right atrium and right ventricle that directs blood flow to the lungs.

V

Valve Regurgitation:
A heart valve problem where blood leaks backward instead of moving forward.

Vasodilator:
A medication that widens blood vessels to reduce blood pressure and help the heart work more easily.

Ventilation / BiPAP / CPAP:
Machines that assist breathing by providing air pressure through a mask, easing strain on the heart and lungs.

W

Weight Monitoring:
Daily weighing to check for fluid buildup — one of the most important tools for managing heart failure.

Appendix A — Preparing for Your Heart Failure Office Visit

What Your Provider Will Ask

Your cardiologist or advanced practice provider (PA or NP) will want to understand **your heart story** — what you've been feeling, when it started, and how it affects your daily life.

Thinking about these questions before your visit can help you feel ready and make your appointment go smoothly.

Symptoms and Changes

□ When did you first notice shortness of breath, swelling, or fatigue?
□ Are your symptoms getting better, worse, or about the same?
□ Do you ever wake up at night short of breath or need extra pillows to sleep?
□ Have you noticed swelling in your feet, ankles, legs, or belly?
□ Do you ever feel your heart racing, skipping beats, or pounding in your chest?
□ Have you gained or lost weight unexpectedly in the past few days or weeks?
□ Do you ever feel dizzy, lightheaded, or more forgetful than usual?

Activity and Daily Living

□ How far can you walk or climb stairs before feeling short of breath or tired?
□ Have you had to stop doing any of your usual activities?
□ How many pillows do you sleep with at night, and can you lie flat comfortably?
□ Are you still able to do your usual chores, or do you need help?

Diet and Fluid Intake

□ How much fluid do you drink in a day?
□ Do you use salt when cooking or at the table?
□ Have you noticed any bloating or loss of appetite?

Medications

□ Are you taking your heart medications exactly as prescribed?
□ Have you missed any doses recently or run out of medication?
□ Do you know the names of your medicines and what they're for?
□ Have you noticed any side effects (dizziness, cough, swelling, etc.)?

Weight and Monitoring

□ Do you weigh yourself every morning?
□ What was your most recent weight change?
□ Do you keep a daily record or use a tracker?

Other Medical History

□ Have you ever been told you had a heart attack or heart valve problem?
□ Do you have high blood pressure, diabetes, or kidney problems?
□ Have you had any recent hospital stays or ER visits for your heart?
□ Does anyone in your family have heart problems or heart failure?

Lifestyle and Support

□ Do you smoke, vape, or drink alcohol?
□ How is your sleep, mood, or stress level lately?
□ Do you live alone or have help at home if you need it?
□ Do you feel safe and able to manage your medications, meals, and doctor visits?

Long-Term Planning

□ Have you discussed your wishes about advanced care (DNR, DNI, living will)?
□ Do you have someone who could make healthcare decisions for you if you couldn't?

Appendix B — Take This to Your First Appointment

Questions to **Ask** Your Heart Provider

- You deserve to understand your diagnosis and care plan.
- Bring this page to your visit and check off the questions you want to ask your cardiologist or advanced practice provider (PA or NP).
- Write notes in the margins or on the back if you need more space.

Understanding Your Diagnosis

□ What type of heart failure do I have — is my heart weak, stiff, or both?
□ What stage or class of heart failure am I in?
□ Can my heart function improve with treatment?
□ Is this something that can get better, or will I always have it?

Treatment and Prognosis

□ Can this be managed with medications alone?
□ What are the goals of my treatment plan?
□ How will we know if my medications are working?
□ Will I need any procedures or surgeries?
□ What can I expect over the next few months or years?

Daily Living

□ What changes should I make to my diet or fluid intake?
□ Is it safe for me to exercise?
□ Should I weigh myself or check my blood pressure at home?
□ Will I need any medical equipment at home (like oxygen or a scale)?
□ What warning signs mean I should call the office or go to the ER?

Support and Planning

□ How often should I follow up with you?
□ Are there support groups or cardiac rehab programs you recommend?
□ Who can I talk to if I need help paying for medications or arranging home care?
□ When should we discuss advance directives or long-term planning?

Tip: *You don't need to ask everything at once. Pick what matters most to you today, and keep this page for future visits.*

Appendix C — Travel Tips

- You can travel safely with heart failure — it just takes a little planning.
- Whether you're driving, flying, or taking a cruise, these steps will help you enjoy your trip while keeping your heart comfortable and protected.

Before You Go

- ☐ **Check with your provider.** Get a quick check-up before long trips to be sure your heart and medications are stable.
- ☐ **Refill prescriptions early.** Bring enough for the trip *plus a few extra days.*
- ☐ **Carry medicines in original bottles** and keep them in your carry-on, not checked luggage.
- ☐ **Pack your medication list,** latest weight record, and provider contact info.
- ☐ **Bring your travel scale** if you'll be gone more than a week.
- ☐ **Wear a medical ID bracelet** or necklace showing you have heart failure.
- ☐ **Ask about travel insurance** if you have advanced disease or frequent flares.

During Car Travel

☐ **Stop every 1–2 hours** to stretch and walk for a few minutes.

☐ **Switch drivers or change positions** to avoid long periods with your legs down.

☐ **Recline slightly or prop legs up** on a small pillow or blanket to reduce swelling.

☐ **Pack low-sodium snacks** and small bottles of water.

☐ **Avoid salty fast food** along the road — choose fruit, nuts, or sandwiches from home.

During Air Travel

☐ **Move your legs often** — flex ankles, wiggle toes, or walk the aisle hourly.

☐ **Ask for an aisle seat** so you can move easily.

☐ **Wear loose clothes and compression socks** (only if your provider approves).

☐ **Keep medications and a light snack** in your carry-on. Airplane meals are usually salty.

☐ **Drink small sips of water** and limit alcohol or caffeine.

- ☐ **If you use oxygen,** contact the airline at least two weeks before your flight for medical clearance.

Hotel or Cruise Tips

- ☐ Request a **room near the elevator** to limit long walks.
- ☐ Use **extra pillows** or a wedge for easier breathing.
- ☐ **Avoid buffets and sauces** — they're high in salt.
- ☐ **Weigh yourself daily** if possible; ask the front desk for a scale.
- ☐ Rest whenever swelling or shortness of breath starts.

When You Return Home

- ☐ Weigh yourself the next morning and compare with your pre-trip weight.
- ☐ Call your provider if you gained **2–3 lb in one day or 5 lb in a week.**
- ☐ Review medications with your pharmacist if you missed or adjusted any doses.
- ☐ Resume your normal diet and routine as soon as you return.

Key Takeaway

- Traveling with heart failure is possible and rewarding — the key is *movement, hydration, and planning*.
- Bring your medications, rest as needed, and monitor your weight.
- Smart travel choices help you see the world while keeping your heart steady and strong.

Monthly Weight Tracker

Date	Weight	UP/DOWN	Notes

Monthly Weight Tracker

Date	Weight	UP/DOWN	Notes

Monthly Weight Tracker

Date	Weight	UP/DOWN	Notes

Monthly Weight Tracker

Date	Weight	UP/DOWN	Notes

Monthly Weight Tracker

Date	Weight	UP/DOWN	Notes

Monthly Weight Tracker

Date	Weight	UP/DOWN	Notes

Quick Index

H

L

M

N

P

Author Note

As a Physician Assistant and educator, my mission is to make medical information clear, compassionate, and truly useful.
Heart Disease 101: A Patient's Complete Guide to Symptoms, Treatments, and Prevention was written to help people understand that heart disease is not the end of the story — it's the start of taking back control through knowledge, prevention, and partnership with your medical team.

This book joins my growing patient education series, which includes *Breast Cancer 101*, *Menopause 101*, and *Osteoporosis 101*, each written to empower patients and families with accurate, evidence-based information they can trust.
Spanish-language editions are also available to reach more North American readers and ensure that vital medical education is accessible to everyone.

Every page in this series is designed for real people — patients, caregivers, and families — who deserve to understand what's happening inside their bodies without feeling lost or overwhelmed.
If these books bring you clarity, comfort, or confidence in your health journey, then they have done their job.

Each book in this series uses trusted U.S. medical guidelines (AHA, ACC, NIH, and Mayo Clinic) and is reviewed periodically for updates to keep information current.

Thank you for reading — and for taking an active role in your health.
You are stronger than you think, inside and out.

— **Stacie the PA**
Duke Residency Trained Physician Assistant
Founder, Medical Things Explained
Author of the Patient Education 101 Series

More Helpful Books by Stacie the PA

Clear, compassionate, and practical guides written by a medical provider who cares.

Hypertension 101

Understand high blood pressure and how to manage it — simply.

Knee Pain 101

From anatomy to treatment options, a complete patient reference.

Hip Pain 101

Everything you need to know about hip pain, diagnosis, and care.

Osteoporosis 101 Defining it and discussing the treatments.

Shoulder Pain 101

An easy-to-follow guide to common shoulder problems and solutions.

Neck Pain 101

A step-by-step look at spine-related neck pain, diagnosis, and treatment options.

Kidney Stones 101

A clear guide to causes, treatments, and prevention strategies.

Pneumonia 101

Learn the basics of prevention, symptoms, and recovery.

Gout 101

Practical answers about causes, flares, and long-term care.

Diverticulosis 101

Understand symptoms, triggers, and treatment of this common digestive condition.

Breast Cancer 101: A Patient's Complete Guide to Symptoms, Treatments, and Prevention

A compassionate, evidence-based guide for patients, survivors, and caregivers — covering everything from diagnosis to recovery and long-term wellness.

Cáncer de Mama 101: Guía Completa para Pacientes

The Spanish-language edition of *Breast Cancer 101* — designed for North

American Spanish-speaking patients and families with the same supportive, educational approach.

✹ **Menopause 101: What Every Husband Should Know About the Change**
A practical guide that bridges understanding and communication between partners.

✹ *Coming Soon: Heart Attack 101, Back Pain 101.*

Check out my website: StaciethePA.com, or find my author page on Amazon: Stacie the PA.

Made in the USA
Monee, IL
04 November 2026

67378704R00105